Practical Math FOR Health Fitness Professionals

Dennis K. Flood, M.S.
Director, Sports Medicine Center
Sarasota Memorial Hospital

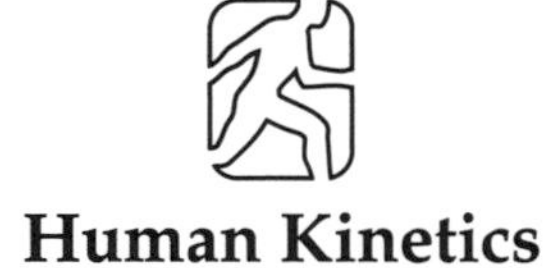

Human Kinetics

Library of Congress Cataloging-in-Publication Data

Flood, Dennis K., 1948–
Practical math for health fitness professionals / Dennis K. Flood.
p. cm.
Includes bibliographical references and index.
ISBN 0-87322-758-1 (pbk.)
1. Exercise--Physiological aspects--Mathematics. 2. Physical therapy--Mathematics. 3. Cardiopulmonary system--Physiology--Mathematics. 4. Sports--Physiological aspects--Mathematics. I. Title.
QP309.F58 1996
612'.044'0151--dc20 95-36602
CIP

ISBN: 0-87322-758-1

Developmental Editor: Holly Gilly; **Assistant Editors:** Ed Giles, Chad Johnson, and Kirby Mittelmeier; **Copyeditor:** Joyce Sexton; **Proofreader:** Sue Fetters; **Indexer:** Theresa Schaefer; **External Content Editor:** Steve Farrell; **Typesetters:** Impressions and Francine Hamerski; **Layout:** Impressions; **Text Designer:** Judy Henderson; **Cover Designer:** Jack Davis; **Photographer:** Derek Khaw; **Illustrator:** Jennifer Delmotte; **Printer:** Edwards Brothers

Human Kinetics books are available at special discounts for bulk purchase. Special editions or book excerpts can also be created to specification. For details, contact the Special Sales Manager at Human Kinetics.

Printed in the United States of America 10 9 8 7 6 5 4 3 2 1

Human Kinetics
P.O. Box 5076, Champaign, IL 61825-5076
1-800-747-4457

Canada: Human Kinetics, Box 24040, Windsor, ON N8Y 4Y9
1-800-465-7301 (in Canada only)

Europe: Human Kinetics, P.O. Box IW14, Leeds LS16 6TR, United Kingdom
(44) 1132 781708

Australia: Human Kinetics, 2 Ingrid Street, Clapham 5062, South Australia
(08) 371 3755

New Zealand: Human Kinetics, P.O. Box 105-231, Auckland 1
(09) 523 3462

Contents

Preface

The purpose of this text is to provide students and practitioners of exercise physiology with the working concepts needed to understand and perform the mathematical calculations required for working with the cardiovascular and respiratory physiological values of subjects who are resting or exercising.

This book can be used in three ways. First, each math problem is built upon the concepts in the previous problem. Basic math leads smoothly into more complex math. An ideal strategy would be to start on the first page of each chapter and progress through each section of the chapter in sequence. By the time you have studied the examples and worked the practice problems, you will have mastered those particular calculations. You may be surprised at the understanding you have gained of this kind of math.

Second, this book can be used as a resource manual for the practitioner already in the field of exercise science. It is a resource for the exercise physiologist, the physical therapist, the nurse working in cardiac or pulmonary rehabilitation, and the physician who is performing routine graded exercise tests, prescribing exercise for patients, and perhaps working in a fitness or athletic setting.

Third, the mathematics throughout these pages can be used as a supplement to the example equations presented in the 1995 American College of Sports Medicine (ACSM) *Guidelines for Exercise Testing and Prescription.*

The chapters in this text are arranged in a specific sequence. The first few chapters introduce the basic concepts and lay a foundation for further work based on these concepts. As you gain a more detailed understanding of these principles in the later chapters, all the pieces begin to fit together.

Chapter 1 is a preview of the major topics in the book. This chapter provides insight into terms and phrases most commonly used in the field of exercise physiology. Chapter 2 reviews the math concepts and tools that are needed in working with math equations in general. The suggestions and information within this chapter will help to alleviate your frustrations with the topic of math.

Chapter 3 introduces the math *unit.* Every math equation is built around mathematical units. When you can manipulate and cancel units, frustrations with math will become enjoyment with math. When you learn to handle math units correctly, you will have much more confidence in your answers.

Chapters 4, 5, and 6 provide the foundation for the math and exercise physiology concepts presented in chapters 7 through 13. Chapters 4, 5, and 6 also include information that is routinely found on exercise physiology exams and in the exercise science literature as well as information and terms that should be a part of the knowledge base of every exercise professional.

Chapters 7 through 13 provide tools, concepts, skills, theory examples, and many practice problems relating to the ACSM metabolic equations that are included on ACSM certification exams.

The explanation of physiology in this book is presented on a basic level. There is no intent to offer detailed explanations of exercise physiology. Rather, the book is a mathematics of physiology primer, intended to pique your curiosity about physiological values and how they are related mathematically. This basic information will provide you with the tools to investigate physiological math relationships that you will encounter elsewhere, such as in other books or in the laboratory in the future. *Physiological concepts* and theories may, and most likely will, change over the years as we learn more and more about exercise physiology. The *math concepts,* on the other hand, will always remain the same.

Special note to students:

In some of the examples and practice problems, more values will be given than are needed to perform the calculations, for three reasons:

1. The additional values given will help you to evaluate and gain a better understanding of the overall context of the problem or situation of the example. The extra values may offer clues for solving the problem.
2. The extra information will also help you to identify the specific values needed to solve the problem and to eliminate those values that are not needed to perform the calculations.
3. While working with the physiological variables in each example and practice problem you will learn how to perform the calculations and also become familiar with the numbers that are related to the variables. For example, you will learn that a glucose value of 190 mg/dl is far above the normal range, that a value of 76 ml O_2/kg/min is an excellent $\dot{V}O_2max$, and that a $\dot{V}E$ of 5 L/min represents a value of someone who is at rest. A list of physiological variables, along with values for trained and untrained individuals, is provided as a resource in Appendix C.

You will find the math straightforward. The methods for solving math problems as outlined within these pages will become your tools for solving math and physiology problems that you encounter in the laboratory, in the field, on the job, and specifically on exams related to exercise physiology.

Dennis K. Flood, M. S.

This text and all of the effort put forth to write these pages are sincerely dedicated to you, who are trying to gain a deeper understanding of the methods for performing fitness-related math. If you are finding the math of physiology frustrating, you will be pleased to know that you are not alone.

These pages were written for you. Use your calculator and follow through the steps for the examples in each chapter. You will enjoy the process and become more confident with the mathematics of exercise physiology.

1 Introduction to Metabolic Mathematics

Major Concepts

Definitions of exercise physiology terms and metabolic math

Basic physiological variables

Direct measurement of $\dot{V}O_2$

Metabolism, metabolic rate, and METs

The main purpose of *Practical Math for Health Fitness Professionals* is to provide you with a working knowledge of physiological variables and the math skills needed to manage the associated values. You will be able to use the math tools to evaluate someone's level of physical fitness, to design an appropriate exercise program, and to identify pathological abnormalities. The metabolic math calculations in this text are the same ones you will encounter on the exams offered by the American College of Sports Medicine (ACSM), the American Council on Exercise (ACE), and other fitness-related institutions.

Basic Definitions

It is important that you understand how the basic terms you'll encounter in this text and on the exams are used and applied.

exercise—Planned, structured, and repetitive bodily movement done to improve or maintain one or more components of physical fitness.

physical activity—Any bodily movement produced by skeletal muscles that results in energy expenditure.*

physical fitness—A set of attributes that people have or achieve that relate to the ability to perform physical activity.*

cardiorespiratory endurance—A health-associated component of physical fitness that relates to the ability of the circulatory and respiratory systems to supply fuel during sustained physical activity and to eliminate fatigue products after supplying fuel.*

muscular strength—A health-associated component of physical fitness that relates to the amount of external force a muscle can exert.*

muscular endurance—A health-associated component of physical fitness that relates to the ability of muscle groups to exert external force for many repetitions or successive exertions.*

ergometer—An exercise device, such as a treadmill, a stationary cycle, a rowing machine, or bench steps, that can be calibrated and set to elicit a specific work requirement.

graded exercise test (GXT)—A test used either as a diagnostic tool or to evaluate the functional capacity of the cardiovascular system. A GXT usually evaluates the physiological response to small increases in work requirement and can be used to measure maximal or submaximal effort.

metabolic math—The manipulation of numbers that represent physiological variables, allowing you to objectively assess fitness and its components. This process is useful to enhance understanding of the interrelationship among physical variables and for the design of appropriate fitness/exercise programs. As you progress through the examples and practice problems in each chapter, you can use Appendix C as a resource for numerical values.

Let's start off with an example of the kind of calculations you will be doing.

Example 1A

Calculate $\dot{Q}$. A male subject is being tested on a stationary bicycle. What is his cardiac output ($\dot{Q}$) if his stroke volume (SV) is 80 ml of blood per beat and his heart rate (HR) is 96 beats per minute? Use the equation: Cardiac output ($\dot{Q}$) = stroke volume (SV) × heart rate (HR).

Step 1: Fill the known values into the equation.

$$\dot{Q} = \frac{80 \text{ ml blood}}{\cancel{\text{beat}}} \times \frac{96\ \cancel{\text{beat}}}{\text{min}}$$

Step 2: Multiply the values.

$$\dot{Q} = \frac{7{,}680 \text{ ml blood}}{\text{min}}$$

The dot over the Q means *per minute.* The two *beat* units cancel each other out, leaving ml blood/min for the answer.

This example illustrates the straightforward approach to math used in this book.

Note.* Definitions are from "Physical Activity, Exercise, and Physical Fitness: Definitions and Distinctions for Health-Related Research" by C. J. Casperson, K. E. Powell, and G. M. Christenson, March–April 1985, *Public Health Reports,* **100, pp. 126–131.

Basic Physiological Variables

As we have already noted, the numbers an exercise physiology professional works with represent a specific set of values, or physiological variables.

Exercise produces many physiological responses. Physiological *changes* occur in response to acute (single bouts of) exercise, and physiological *adaptations* occur in response to repeated exercise sessions, closely spaced over time (e.g., three to six times a week for 6 weeks). Some of the basic variables that change with exercise (definitions of the terms appear in the glossary) are volume of oxygen consumed in 1 min, minute ventilation, blood pressure, heart rate, arteriovenous difference, frequency of breaths per minute, tidal volume, stroke volume, cardiac output in 1 min, and metabolic equivalents. By understanding the mathematics behind the physiological variables that relate to exercise physiology, you will be able to

- follow an individual's progress over a period of exercise training,
- determine the maximal response to exercise effort,
- prescribe the appropriate intensity of exercise for training sessions,
- determine the workload that someone is presently training at, and,
- in an individual with cardiorespiratory or metabolic disease, possibly determine the site (heart, lungs, or muscle) that is limiting exercise tolerance.

Introduction to Oxygen Consumption

Since the 1950s oxygen uptake, or oxygen consumption, has been used to define aerobic fitness. Because aerobic fitness is the foundation of a fitness assessment, it is necessary for the exercise professional to be able to determine an individual's submaximal (submax) oxygen consumption as well as oxygen consumption at the physiological upper limits of exercise ($\dot{V}O_2max$).

The direct method for determining oxygen consumption is the most objective. The way to measure O_2 consumption ($\dot{V}O_2$) directly is to collect and analyze expired gases by using methods of open-circuit spirometry, through which quantity data are collected in one of two ways, depending on the type of system used. Some systems collect expired gases in Douglas bags during each 2- to 3-min stage of an exercise test, analyzing the mixed sample from each bag. Other systems measure O_2 and CO_2 values breath by breath. Each breath is analyzed for its content of oxygen, carbon dioxide, and nitrogen. Both systems have advantages and disadvantages (Froelicher, 1989; Jones, 1988; McArdle, Katch, & Katch, 1994; Wasserman, Hansen, Sue, & Whipp, 1987). $\dot{V}O_2$ can also be estimated based on physical response to a standardized workload.

Introduction to Metabolism

The term metabolism is used often, but few have a good grasp of what metabolism really represents. Metabolism, or metabolic rate, is the rate at which the body consumes oxygen and produces energy in the form of adenosine triphosphate (ATP). In general the metabolic rate is highest during intense exercise and lowest during restful sleep. Body size, age, type of food intake, level of activity, thyroid hormone levels, and the ratio of body fat to lean tissue all affect metabolic rate.

At rest, the average person's metabolism is about 1 metabolic equivalent (MET), approximately 3.5 ml O_2/kg/min (each kilogram of body weight is using 3.5 ml of

O_2 per minute). An endurance athlete may have a resting MET level near 3.5 (such as 3.6 to 4.0 ml O_2/kg/min), while a very sedentary individual with a relatively high percentage of body fat and a lower lean (muscle) tissue ratio may have a resting MET level below 3.5 (such as 3.2 to 3.4 ml O_2/kg/min).

A number of examples and practice problems in this book involve calculations dealing with body weight, body composition, metabolism, and MET levels. The value of 3.5 ml O_2/kg/min will represent 1 MET in all of these calculations. When you are working with MET levels, you must think of METs as multiples of resting metabolism. Five METs, for example, represents a level of activity that is five times above resting metabolism. Nine METs is an energy expenditure that is nine times above resting, and so on.

Summary

More exercise professionals are working in a wider variety of exercise-related fields than ever before. Professionals are testing and writing exercise prescriptions for patients who have heart disease, lung disease, and other physical and metabolic disorders. Exercise professionals are also being asked to work with astronauts and pilots, professional race car drivers, and individuals with mental and physical disabilities. They are doing testing and training for deep sea divers and prescribing exercise for women before and after childbirth. To work successfully with this wide diversity of groups, exercise professionals need to be able to properly conduct assessments of aerobic capacity and perform the related calculations to convert the raw data into a useful form. This book will help you gain the confidence and skills and give you the tools to perform almost any exercise physiology math problem that you encounter.

Understanding metabolic calculations is an excellent way to gain an understanding of the nuts and bolts of exercise physiology and a depth of comprehension into the field of exercise science.

Chapters 2 and 3 are important as preparation for the other chapters in this book. To gain the most benefit from this text, do not bypass the vital information presented within these next two chapters.

2 Review of General Math

Major Concepts

Multiplication
Division
Working with fractions and decimals
Solving algebraic equations

In writing this textbook I assume that you know basic math concepts. This chapter reviews specific math functions that you will need to understand the metabolic calculations to come. If you find that you need more review of your math skills, you can refer to any basic math book. A review of basic algebra concepts can be found in Pulsinelli and Hooper (1987).

Multiplication

Multiplication is the process of adding the same number several times. For example, 4 times 2 means $2 + 2 + 2 + 2$, or $4 \times 2 = 8$.

There are various ways of expressing multiplication, such as a times b.

$$ab \qquad a \times b \qquad a \cdot b \qquad a(b) \qquad (a)(b)$$

In this book you will see all of these ways used to multiply numbers, but the $\times$ for multiplication will be used most often. So, for example, when $a = 5$ and $b = 4$, $a \times b = 20$ ($5 \times 4 = 20$). You will also see parentheses used, as in $(3)(6) = 18$.

The answer to a multiplication problem is called the *product.* In the problem $5 \times 4 = 20$, the number 20 is the product of 5 and 4.

Division

Division means the number of times that one number fits into another. For example, 5 fits into 35 seven times, or $35 \div 5 = 7$. The answer resulting from a division problem is called the *quotient* (in this case, 7).

There are various ways to express division:

$$\frac{a}{b} = \qquad a/b = \qquad a \div b =$$

The first two expressions will be used most often in this book. If $a = 15$ and $b = 3$, $\frac{a}{b} = \frac{15}{3} = 5$ (3 fits into 15 five times).

The slanted division sign (/) also means *per,* as used in the expression miles per hour (miles/hr, or mph). The *per* also relates to division. If we were walking at 4 mph we could fit 4 miles into 1 hr. Another example is 12 breaths/minute: 12 breaths are occurring within 1 minute. Twelve is the number, and breaths/minute is the unit.

The unit, meters per minute, abbreviated m/min, will also be used often throughout this book. The slanted line (/) means division, as in the walking speed, 98 m/min. This is 98 m traveled in 1 min.

Working With Fractions and Decimals

A fraction is an expression of division, one term divided by another, yielding a decimal. The top number of a fraction is called the numerator. The bottom number is called the denominator. To convert a fraction to a decimal, simply divide the numerator by the denominator: For example, $100/25 = 4$, $100/8 = 12.5$, and $100/3 = 33.333$. When a fraction is inverted the numerator and the denominator switch places. Inverting a fraction, especially when doing certain division problems, will significantly simplify the math process of a problem. Inversion changes the value of the quotient of the fraction; for example, $25/100 = 1/4$ when inverted becomes $100/25 = 4$.

Rounding Off Decimals

In this text we will round off final answers to two places to the right of the decimal point.

1st place (the tenths place)
2nd place (the hundredths place)
3rd place (the thousandths place)

93.123 yd

In performing a series of math calculations you should leave the decimal *as is* until you are finished. When you have arrived at the final answer, then round off the number to two places to the right of the decimal.

It is assumed that the reader has knowledge of rounding off numbers. Any general mathematics textbook will provide further review.

Reducing a Fraction to Its Lowest Terms

When the numerator and denominator of a fraction cannot both be divided by the same number (other than 1), the fraction is said to be in its lowest terms. For example, the fraction 5/6 is in its lowest terms because you cannot divide *both* the numerator and the denominator by any number other than 1. The fraction 12/15 is not in its lowest terms because you can divide both numerator and denominator by 3. When this division is performed, the fraction 12/15 is reduced to 4/5. Other examples of fractions reduced to the lowest terms are 6/8 = 3/4, 12/14 = 6/7, and 21/27 = 7/9.

Multiplication of Fractions

Multiplying fractions is straightforward. The numerators are multiplied together to get the numerator part of the answer, and the denominators are multiplied together to get the denominator of the answer.

Example 2A

Multiply fractions.

$$\frac{5}{6} \times \frac{2}{3} =$$

Step 1: Multiply the numerators and denominators.

$$\frac{5}{6} \times \frac{2}{3} = \frac{10}{18}$$

Step 2: Reduce to the lowest terms.

$$\frac{10}{18} = \frac{5}{9}$$

Dividing Fractions

When the numerator *and* the denominator in a problem are both fractions, inverting the denominator turns a complex division problem into a simple multiplication process. Example 2B shows how to divide one fraction by another fraction. You will use this technique when doing calculations relating to the arm ergometer and the cycle ergometer.

Example 2B

Divide one fraction by another.

$$\frac{2}{3} \div \frac{4}{5} = \text{ or } \frac{\frac{2}{3}}{\frac{4}{5}}$$

Step 1: Simply invert the $\frac{4}{5}$ to $\frac{5}{4}$.

Step 2: Multiply.

$$\frac{2}{3} \times \frac{5}{4} = \frac{10}{12}$$

Step 3: Reduce.

$$\frac{10}{12} = \frac{5}{6}$$

Adding and Subtracting Fractions When the Denominators Are the Same

When adding or subtracting fractions, if the denominators are the same, simply carry the denominator over to the answer. The numerators then can be added or subtracted.

Example 2C

Add fractions when the denominators are the same.

Step 1: Read the problem.

$$\frac{3}{8} + \frac{4}{8} =$$

Step 2: Transfer the denominator over.

$$\frac{3}{8} + \frac{4}{8} = \frac{}{8}$$

Step 3: Add the numerators.

$$\frac{3}{8} + \frac{4}{8} = \frac{7}{8}$$

We will use this concept when doing calculations to determine $\dot{V}O_2$ on the cycle ergometer and arm ergometer.

Example 2D

Subtract fractions when the denominators are the same.

Step 1: Read the problem.

$$\frac{5}{7} - \frac{2}{7} =$$

Step 2: Carry the denominator over.

$$\frac{5}{7} - \frac{2}{7} = \frac{}{7}$$

Step 3: Subtract.

$$\frac{5}{7} - \frac{2}{7} = \frac{3}{7}$$

We do not need to consider adding and subtracting fractions that have different denominators. This situation does not arise in physiological math. If you would like additional information about adding and subtracting fractions, you can refer to any basic math textbook.

Cancellation of Terms in Working With Fractions

The process of *cancellation* can be done only when you are performing multiplication or division. Cancellation lets you make a complex math problem more manageable by reducing the size of the numbers.

Here is a multiplication problem done without canceling:

$$\frac{1}{3} \times \frac{6}{2} \times \frac{2}{4} \times \frac{4}{6} = \frac{48}{144} = \frac{1}{3}$$

The number 48 divides into 48 one time and into 144 three times, yielding 1/3. In the example that follows, we will use canceling to make this problem easier.

Example 2E

Use canceling to multiply fractions.

Step 1: Look for pairs of like terms (the same term appearing in one of the numerators and one of the denominators). You can cancel these.

$$\frac{1}{3} \times \frac{\cancel{6}}{\cancel{2}} \times \frac{\cancel{2}}{\cancel{4}} \times \frac{\cancel{4}}{\cancel{6}} =$$

Step 2: Solve with the remaining terms.

$$\frac{1}{3} = \frac{1}{3}$$

The 6's cancel each other, the 4's cancel each other, and the 2's cancel each other. And the result in this case is that you end up not having to do any calculation at all. Cancellation reduces problems down to their lowest terms; always use it to make problems easier to perform. Remember that you cancel only when multiplying and dividing fractions.

Example 2F shows a combination of math principles in which a fraction divided by another fraction is converted into a multiplication problem.

Example 2F

Combine math techniques. We start with a division problem, convert it into a multiplication problem, perform the process of cancellation, and then multiply, yielding a product at it lowest terms.

Step 1: Read the problem.

$$\frac{\frac{2}{3}}{\frac{4}{5}} =$$

Step 2: Invert the fraction in the denominator. It is now a multiplier.

$$\frac{2}{3} \times \frac{5}{4} =$$

Step 3: Cancel and solve.

$$\frac{{}^{1}\not{2}}{3} \times \frac{5}{\not{4}_{2}} = \frac{5}{6}$$

Adding and Subtracting Decimals

The first step in preparing to add or subtract decimals is to line up the decimal points in the same column, as shown in examples 2G and 2H. Then proceed to add or subtract the numbers.

Example 2G

Add decimals. Add the three components of the treadmill walking equation to calculate total oxygen consumption ($\dot{V}O_2$) (you will learn more about this in chapter 8). The number that represents each of the three $\dot{V}O_2$ components is a decimal. Each decimal is followed by its unit, i.e., ml of O_2/kg/min. In this problem, the horizontal component is 5.36 ml O_2/kg/min, the vertical component is 1.93 ml/O_2/kg/min, and the resting component is 3.5 ml O_2/kg/min. To add numbers together all of the units must be the same.

Horizontal component		Vertical component		Rest component
5.36 ml O_2/kg/min	+	1.93 ml O_2/kg/min	+	3.5 ml O_2/kg/min

Step 1: Line up the decimal points into a straight column.

	Horiz	5.36 ml O_2/kg/min
	Vert	1.93 ml O_2/kg/min
	+ Rest	3.50 ml O_2/kg/min
Total $\dot{V}O_2$ =		

Step 2: Add all of the components together to get the total $\dot{V}O_2$.

	Horiz	5.36 ml O_2/kg/min
	Vert	1.93 ml O_2/kg/min
	+ Rest	3.50 ml O_2/kg/min
Total $\dot{V}O_2$ =		10.79 ml O_2/kg/min

Example 2H

Subtract decimals. Subtract 4.23 from 6.31.

Step 1: Align the decimals.

Step 2: Subtract and solve.

$$\begin{array}{r} 6.31 \\ -\ 4.23 \\ \hline 2.08 \end{array}$$

Solving Algebraic Equations

The term *algebraic equation* means *a series of basic and common mathematical functions.* It is important to understand algebraic equations in order to perform calculations dealing with the treadmill, cycle, arm crank, and stair stepping.

Two steps are involved in solving an algebraic equation. The first step is to identify the units that you want the answer to be in. Suppose, for example, we want to convert mph to m/min. We want the answer to be in the unit m/min.

When 3 mph is converted to m/min the units mph cancel each other out, leaving m/min as the answer. The multiplication yields the number 80.4.

$$3 \cancel{\text{mph}} \times \frac{26.8 \text{ m/min}}{1 \cancel{\text{mph}}} = 80.4 \text{ m/min}$$

The concept of units will be discussed in more detail in chapter 3.

The second step, and the most important one for performing algebraic equations, is to *isolate the desired unit on one side of the equation.* In the first step we identified the unit we wanted the answer to be in as m/min; then we placed the m/min by itself on the right side of the equation (the right side of the = sign).

In Examples 2I, J, and K we isolate the unit we want in a very simple equation, $a = \frac{b}{c}$.

Example 2I

Solve for *a*.

$$b = 15, c = 5$$

Step 1: Read the equation.

$$a = \frac{b}{c}$$

Step 2: Plug in the numbers, divide, and solve.

$$a = \frac{15}{5} \qquad a = 3$$

It was easy to solve for a because a was already isolated on the left side of the = sign.

Example 2J

Solve for *b*.

$$c = 5, a = 3$$

Step 1: Read the equation.

$$a = \frac{b}{c}$$

Step 2: Isolate b by multiplying both sides of the equation by c.

$$(c)a = \frac{b(c)}{c}$$

Step 3: Cancel the top and bottom c on the right side.

$$(c)a = \frac{b\cancel{(c)}}{\cancel{c}}$$

Step 4: Plug in the numbers, multiply, and solve.

$(5)3 = b \qquad b = 15$

Example 2K

Solve for *c*.

$b = 15, a = 3$

Step 1: Read the equation.

$$a = \frac{b}{c}$$

Step 2: Isolate c by multiplying both sides of the equation by $\frac{c}{a}$.

$$\frac{ca}{a} = \frac{cb}{ac}$$

Step 3: Cancel each c and each a.

$$\frac{c\cancel{a}}{\cancel{a}} = \frac{\cancel{c}b}{a\cancel{c}}$$

Step 4: Plug in the numbers, divide, and solve.

$c = \frac{15}{3} \qquad c = 5$

To find the right combination in order to isolate a unit may require some trial and error. With practice you will be able to isolate the correct unit so that the algebraic equation can be solved easily. Examples 2L and 2M provide more practice.

Example 2L

Solve for *a*.

$c = 3, b = 4, \text{ml} = 2$

Step 1: Read the equation.

$$\frac{a}{b} = \frac{c}{\text{ml}}$$

Step 2: Multiply both sides of the equation by b to isolate a. Cancel.

$$\frac{(b)a}{b} = \frac{c(b)}{\text{ml}}$$

Step 3: Plug in the numbers and solve.

$$a = \frac{3(4)}{2}$$
$$a = 6$$

Example 2M

Convert 6 ft to the unit *inches.* This is an illustration of reducing a problem to its lowest terms as well as canceling units to identify the desired unit for the answer.

Step 1: Identify the desired unit for the answer.

The desired unit for the answer is *inches.*

Step 2: Determine how many inches in one foot.

The conversion factor is 12 in = 1 ft.

Step 3: Set up the equation.

The feet cancel each other out, leaving inches as the unit for the answer.

$$6 \text{ ft} \times \frac{12 \text{ in}}{1 \text{ ft}} = ? \text{ in}$$

Step 4: Perform the math.

$$6 \text{ ft} \times \frac{12 \text{ in}}{1 \text{ ft}} = 72 \text{ in}$$

Temperature Conversion Equations

Temperature conversion is an application of some of the basic manipulations we have reviewed. When you know °C (degrees Celsius), you can find °F (degrees Fahrenheit) using this equation: °F = (1.8 × °C) + 32. As a rule in mathematics, the calculation within the parentheses is performed first. For example, when °C = 50:

$$°F = (1.8 \times °C) + 32$$
$$°F = (1.8 \times 50) + 32$$
$$°F = (90) + 32$$
$$°F = 122$$

So 50 °C is equal to 122 °F.

To convert °F to °C, use this equation:

$$°C = \frac{(°F - 32)}{1.8}$$

For example, when °F = 59,

$$°C = \frac{(59 - 32)}{1.8}$$

So 59 °F is equal to 15 °C.

As you work through the walking, running, stepping, cycling, and arm ergometer equations in the following chapters, you will recognize how the examples you have seen so far apply to solving those math problems.

Summary

In this chapter we have reviewed multiplication and division of whole numbers and fractions and looked briefly at adding and subtracting decimals. There was a review of the important process of isolating a unit in order to solve an algebraic equation. The term *unit* was introduced in a few examples. The unit is an important concept. Keeping close track of the units while doing a math problem is the key for successfully performing physiological math. The unit will be explored in more detail in chapter 3.

Proceed to the practice problems. You will notice that in problems 3, 4, and 5, each number is followed by its unit. The answers will follow the series of practice problems.

Chapter 2 Practice Problems

The answers for problems throughout the book are given on the pages following the problems.

1. Complete the following. Divide one fraction by another.

   (a) $\frac{2}{3} \div \frac{1}{4} =$

   (b) $\frac{7}{8} \div \frac{3}{4} =$

   (c) Divide the fraction 5/6 by the fraction 1/8.
   $$\frac{\frac{5}{6}}{\frac{1}{8}}$$

   (d) Divide the fraction 7/8 by the fraction 2/1.
   $$\frac{\frac{7}{8}}{\frac{2}{1}}$$

2. Add these fractions.

   (a) $\frac{7}{8} + \frac{5}{8} =$

(b) $\frac{2}{3} + \frac{1}{3} =$

(c) $\frac{1}{4} + \frac{2}{4} =$

3. Round off the following numbers to two places to the right of the decimal point. Write out each number with its unit.

(a) 1.263 kg

(b) 23.04193 ml O_2

(c) 23.46828 m/min

(d) 18.998 ml O_2/kg/min

4. Use the Fahrenheit equation to convert the following Celsius temperatures to degrees Fahrenheit.

(a) 37 °C

(b) −15 °C

5. Use the Celsius equation to convert Fahrenheit temperature to degrees Celsius.

(a) 100 °F

(b) 6 °F

Chapter 2 Answers to Practice Problems

1. All answers are reduced to lowest terms and converted to a decimal.

(a) $\frac{2}{3} \times \frac{4}{1} = \frac{8}{3}$ or 2 and 2/3 = 2.67

(b) $\frac{7}{8} \times \frac{4}{3} = \frac{28}{24} = \frac{7}{6}$ = 1 and 4/24 or 1 and 1/6 = 1.17

(c) $\frac{5}{6} \times \frac{8}{1} = \frac{40}{6} = \frac{20}{3}$ = 6 and 4/6 or 6 and 2/3 = 6.67

(d) $\frac{7}{8} \times \frac{1}{2} = \frac{7}{16}$ = 0.4375, rounded off to 0.44

2. All answers are reduced to lowest terms and converted to a decimal.

(a) $\frac{12}{8} = \frac{3}{2}$ = 1 and 4/8 or 1 and 1/2 = 1.50

(b) 3/3 = 1.00

(c) 3/4 = 0.75
(Writing a decimal as .75 and as 0.75 are both acceptable.)

3. Rounding off decimals to two places

(a) 1.26 kg

(b) 23.04 ml O_2

(c) 23.47 m/min

(d) 19.00 ml O_2/kg/min

4. Fahrenheit

   (a) 98.6 °F

   (b) 5 °F

5. Celsius

   (a) 37.78 °C

   (b) −14.44 °C

3 Mathematical Units and Problem Solving

Major Concepts

Mathematical units

Cancellation of units

Conversion factors

The math symbol X^{-1}

One of the most challenging areas for students of exercise physiology is solving mathematical problems. Exercise physiology deals exclusively with measurable quantities. Table 3.1 provides an abbreviated list of measurable quantities called *units of measure.* From this point forward we will refer to units of measure as a *unit.* In order to fully understand the concepts and principles of exercise physiology you must have an understanding of both the numbers and the units used in this field.

The problems you will encounter in this chapter will be slightly more difficult than those in chapter 2. Upon completion of this chapter you will be able to use

Table 3.1 Units of Measure

Length	inch, foot, yard, mile, centimeter, meter, kilometer
Volume	ounce, quart, gallon, milliliters, liters
Mass	ounce, pound, gram, kilogram
Time	second, minute, hour
Energy	calorie, kilocalorie ml O_2/kg/min, ml O_2/min, Watts, newtons, kilopond-meters, METs

units and conversion factors as tools to successfully complete exercise physiology–related math problems.

The Unit

Numbers without their unit of measure have little meaning in exercise physiology. For example, take the number 325. If 325 is the number of pounds (units) that a football player weighs, the number has meaning. This is a big football player. Thus, all numbers that represent measurement must be labeled with the proper unit (ft, lb, min, etc.) to be meaningful and useful. A complete list of units and their abbreviations can be found in Appendix A.

You can use units to confirm the answers to math problems. In Example 3A, follow the units along through the problem. You will notice that the unit that does not cancel out is the correct unit for the answer. If you examine the process carefully you will find it valuable for understanding how units are used and how the cancellation process works to make math problems manageable. In most problems, as you will see, only one conversion factor is used at a time.

Example 3A

Convert yards to meters. The problem is stated using only the units.

Step 1: Read the problem.

$$\text{yd} \times \frac{\text{ft}}{\text{yd}} \times \frac{\text{in}}{\text{ft}} \times \frac{\text{cm}}{\text{in}} \times \frac{\text{m}}{\text{cm}} =$$

Step 2: Cancel.

$$\cancel{\text{yd}} \times \frac{\cancel{\text{ft}}}{\cancel{\text{yd}}} \times \frac{\cancel{\text{in}}}{\cancel{\text{ft}}} \times \frac{\cancel{\text{cm}}}{\cancel{\text{in}}} \times \frac{\text{m}}{\cancel{\text{cm}}} = \text{m}$$

The unit in the numerator (top) cancels out the same unit in the denominator (bottom). The only unit not canceled out is the meter (m); therefore, meters is the unit for the answer.

Step 3: Add numbers to the units.

$$10\ \cancel{\text{yd}} \times \frac{3\ \cancel{\text{ft}}}{1\ \cancel{\text{yd}}} \times \frac{12\ \cancel{\text{in}}}{1\ \cancel{\text{ft}}} \times \frac{2.54\ \cancel{\text{cm}}}{1\ \cancel{\text{in}}} \times \frac{1\ \text{m}}{100\ \cancel{\text{cm}}} = 9.14\ \text{m}$$

Cancel the units and multiply and divide the numbers.

This process of canceling eliminates confusion, confirming that the unit for the answer is meters and not inches, feet, yards, or centimeters. The process of cancellation also ensures that the numbers are multiplied or divided correctly and in the proper order. *Each of the fractions in step 3 is a conversion factor.* Conversion factors will be discussed in more detail in the next section of this chapter.

The foregoing example illustrates a rule of thumb for the solution of exercise physiology math problems:

➤ When the unit(s) is correct at the end of a problem, you will be certain that the answer, in number form, is also correct.

This rule is the key to this entire textbook. When the units are correct, the answer will be correct, providing of course, that all of the units are handled and canceled properly and the arithmetic is performed without error. Remembering this can be especially helpful in a situation such as an ACSM exam, where knowing the correct units enables you to confirm your answer to a multiple choice question.

Conversion Factors

A conversion factor is a tool used to convert one unit to another unit. All conversion factors must equal 1. The conversion factor, 12 in = 1 ft, used in Example 3A, equals 1; 1 ft is the same distance as 12 in. The equation 2 ft = 24 in can also be used as a conversion factor.

Another example of a conversion factor is 26.8 m/min = 1 mph. The two values are the same speed. Again, 1 L = 1,000 ml is a conversion factor. These two values are the same quantity.

Sometimes a conversion factor will be written as follows:

$$\frac{454\text{ g}}{1\text{ lb}} = 1 \text{ or } \frac{1\text{ lb}}{454\text{ g}} = 1$$

The number 1 following the conversion factor means that both values are the same weight, distance, volume, quantity, etc. The number 1 does not have a unit. A conversion factor must equal 1. If it does not equal 1 it is not a conversion factor. See Appendix B for an extensive list of conversion factors.

Exercise physiology deals extensively with the conversion of one unit to another unit. In example 3A, yards were converted to meters: 10 yd = 9.14 m. Units are canceled mathematically just as though they were numbers.

Example 3B

Convert feet (ft) to inches (in). You have been asked to convert 5 ft into inches.

Step 1: Determine the conversion factor.
You know that 1 ft = 12 in. The conversion factor 1 ft = 12 in can be expressed in two ways: 1 ft/12 in = 1 or 12 in/1 ft = 1.

The two ways of expressing this conversion factor are essentially the same; one is just the inversion of the other. Which form of this conversion factor should be used to solve the problem of converting feet to inches? The unit that we want in our answer is *inches*. And we want the units of feet to cancel out. The conversion factor that we need to use has feet in the denominator (bottom) position. We will then choose the conversion factor that has the unit *inches on the top*, in the numerator position.

Step 2: Set up the equation.

$$5\text{ ft} \times \frac{12\text{ in}}{1\text{ ft}} =$$

Step 3: Cancel and multiply.

$$5\,\cancel{\text{ft}} \times \frac{12\text{ in}}{1\,\cancel{\text{ft}}} = 60\text{ in}$$

The unit *ft* cancels, leaving the unit *in* as the answer.

As you work through the following examples, you will find it helpful to write each problem down. Cancel the units as you go along and examine how each conversion factor is used to solve the problem. Your confidence level when working with this type of math will improve.

Example 3C

Convert inches to centimeters.

Step 1: Determine the conversion factor.

$$\text{in} \times \frac{\text{cm}}{\text{in}} =$$

The conversion factor is cm/in.

Step 2: Cancel and multiply.

$$\cancel{\text{in}} \times \frac{\text{cm}}{\cancel{\text{in}}} = \text{cm}$$

The inches cancel each other out. The unit *cm* is the answer.

Example 3D

Convert 4 mph to m/min.

Step 1: Determine the conversion factor.
In this case, the conversion factor can be:

$$\frac{26.8 \text{ m/min}}{1 \text{ mph}} = 1 \text{ or } \frac{1 \text{ mph}}{26.8 \text{ m/min}} = 1$$

The conversion factor that must be used is the one that has the unit for the answer in the top position. The unit for the answer is m/min.

Step 2: Set up the equation.

$$4 \text{ mph} \times \frac{26.8 \text{ m/min}}{1 \text{ mph}} =$$

Step 3: Solve.

$$4 \cancel{\text{mph}} \times \frac{26.8 \text{ m/min}}{1 \cancel{\text{mph}}} = 107.2 \text{ m/min}$$

The units *mph* cancel each other. The *m/min* remains uncanceled as the answer.

Make sure that you memorize this conversion factor:

$$\frac{26.8 \text{ m/min}}{1 \text{ mph}}$$

You will need to use this conversion factor in every walking and running equation. You should also know that speeds below 4 mph are walking speeds and speeds of 4 mph and above are running speeds.

Example 3E

Convert 75 m/min to ml O_2/kg/min.

Step 1: Determine the conversion factor.

$$\frac{\text{m/min}}{0.1 \text{ ml } O_2\text{/kg/min}} \text{ or } \frac{0.1 \text{ ml } O_2\text{/kg/min}}{\text{m/min}}$$

Step 2: Set up the equation and solve.

$$75 \cancel{\text{m/min}} \times \frac{0.1 \text{ ml } O_2\text{/kg/min}}{\cancel{\text{m/min}}} = 7.5 \text{ ml } O_2\text{/kg/min}$$

In chapter 7 you will be using this conversion often when calculating the walking equation for determining total $\dot{V}O_2$. The conversion that we performed in Example 3E is actually the horizontal component of the treadmill walking equation.

Example 3F

Convert $\frac{4{,}000 \text{ ml } O_2}{\text{min}}$ to $\frac{\text{kcal}}{\text{min}}$.

Step 1: Determine the conversion factor.
The conversion factor is .005 kcal/1 ml O_2.
The number 1 in the denominator is optional. When the unit is written ml O_2, 1 ml of O_2 is assumed. You will often see units expressed without the number 1: .005 kcal/ml O_2, for example.

Step 2: Set up the equation and solve.

$$\frac{4{,}000 \cancel{\text{ml } O_2}}{1 \text{ min}} \times \frac{.005 \text{ kcal}}{\cancel{\text{ml } O_2}} = \frac{20 \text{ kcal}}{1 \text{ min}} \text{ (also can be written 20 kcal/min)}$$

Example 3G

Convert 5 METs to ml O_2/kg/min.

Step 1: Determine the conversion factor.

$$\frac{3.5 \text{ ml } O_2\text{/kg/min}}{1 \text{ MET}}$$

Step 2: Set up the equation and solve.

$$5 \cancel{\text{METs}} \times \frac{3.5 \text{ ml } O_2\text{/kg/min}}{1 \cancel{\text{MET}}} = 17.5 \text{ ml } O_2\text{/kg/min}$$

To summarize, a subject who is working at 5 METs is consuming 17.5 ml O_2/kg/min.

The conversion process in this example is used so often in exercise physiology that it should be memorized: 1 MET = 3.5 ml O_2/kg/min.

Example 3H includes three steps with added complexity. The values, units, and calculations in this example are an introduction to the type of problems that you will be seeing throughout the following chapters.

Example 3H

Determine kcal when you know ml O_2/kg/min. Hal Jones, who weighs 150 lb, is walking on a treadmill at an intensity of 5 METs and is consuming 17.5 ml O_2/kg/min. Determine the number of kcal of energy Hal is using during each minute of walking.

Step 1: Convert the subject's weight in lb to kg.

$$150 \not{\text{lb}} \times \frac{1\text{ kg}}{2.2 \not{\text{lb}}} = 68\text{ kg}$$

Step 2: Using 68 kg of body weight, convert the $\dot{V}O_2$ of 17.5 ml O_2/kg/min to ml/O_2.
(See the glossary for definitions of relative $\dot{V}O_2$ and absolute $\dot{V}O_2$.)

(Relative $\dot{V}O_2$) (Absolute $\dot{V}O_2$)

$$68 \not{\text{kg}} \times \frac{17.5\text{ ml }O_2}{\not{\text{kg}}/\text{min}} = 1{,}190\text{ ml }O_2/\text{min}$$

Step 3: Convert the $\frac{1{,}190\text{ ml }O_2}{\text{min}}$ to $\frac{\text{kcal}}{\text{min}}$.

$$\frac{1{,}190 \not{\text{ml }O_2}}{\text{min}} \times \frac{.005\text{ kcal}}{\not{\text{ml }O_2}} = \frac{5.95\text{ kcal}}{1\text{ min}}$$

At 5 METs Hal is consuming almost 6 kcal of energy per minute while walking on the treadmill. This would be true for any 150-lb subject at this level of intensity.

For practice, perform this calculation using a subject who weighs 165 lb, then one who weighs 102 kg.

The Math Symbol X^{-1}

As you read about various physiology topics, you will come across the symbol of X^{-1}. The X represents any number or unit. This notation, designed to save space, can be confusing at first. The notation $^{-1}$ means to place the number or unit under the division line. So, for example, the notation 6 L · min^{-1} means the same thing as 6 L/min. By eliminating the $^{-1}$ notation you can set up a math problem so that the units conveniently cancel and the numbers become easier to multiply or divide.

Here are some other examples of the $^{-1}$ notation and its alternate form:

Scientific notation		Usable form
sec^{-1}	=	1/sec or $\frac{1}{\text{sec}}$
$\text{N} \cdot \text{m} \cdot \text{sec}^{-1}$	=	$\frac{\text{N} \times \text{m}}{\text{sec}}$

$25\ ml\ O_2 \cdot kg^{-1} \cdot min^{-1}$	=	$25\ ml\ O_2/kg/min$
$100\ m \cdot min^{-1}$	=	$100\ m/min$

Progress to the next section, which has practice problems like the examples in this chapter.

Chapter 3 Practice Problems

Conversion factors are listed in Appendix B.

1. Convert 100 yd to units of feet.

   Use $\frac{3\ ft}{1\ yd}$ as the conversion factor.

2. Convert 300 ft to units of inches.

   Which conversion factor must be used?
   Use $\frac{12\ in}{1\ ft}$ or $\frac{1\ ft}{12\ in}$.

3. Convert 3,600 in to centimeters.

   Use $\frac{1\ in}{2.54\ cm}$ as the conversion factor.

4. Convert 9,144 cm to meters.

   Use $\frac{1\ m}{100\ cm}$.

You have just converted yards to meters as you progressed from problems 1 through 4: 100 yd = 91.44 m. This can be reduced to lowest terms as 1 yd = .914 m or 1 yd/.914 m, which is the conversion factor for directly converting yards to meters, or meters to yards.

5. Convert 5 miles to kilometers. Which conversion factor must be used?

   $\frac{1\ mile}{1.62\ km}$ or $\frac{1.62\ km}{1\ mile}$

6. A walker covers 1 mile in 25 min. How many miles per hour is he walking?

   You are asked to convert $\frac{1\ mile}{25\ min}$ to $\frac{mile}{hr}$. Use $\frac{60\ min}{1\ hr}$.

7. Convert 2.4 mph to m/min.

   Use $\frac{26.8\ m/min}{mph}$ as the conversion factor.

8. Convert the following mph to units of m/min.

   (a) Walking 3.1 mph

   (b) Walking 3.70 mph

   (c) Running 7.5 mph

9. Convert the following m/min to mph. Label each of your answers as walking or running.
   (a) 57 m/min
   (b) 67 m/min
   (c) 147.40 m/min
10. For an 80-kg man, determine kcal/min using the following relative $\dot{V}O_2$ values.
   (a) 20 ml O_2/kg/min
   (b) 32 ml O_2/kg/min
   Hints: (1) Write down the units every time.
   (2) $\frac{\text{ml } O_2}{\text{kg/min}} \times \text{kg} \times \frac{.005 \text{ kcal}}{\text{ml } O_2} =$
   (3) The kg cancel and the ml O_2 cancel.
11. Determine the kcal/min using the following absolute $\dot{V}O_2$ values. (An absolute $\dot{V}O_2$ is a value not including the subject's weight.)
   (a) 1,920 ml O_2/min
   (b) 2,200 ml O_2/min
   (c) 6,080 ml O_2/min (This absolute $\dot{V}O_2$ value represents the value of a world-class endurance athlete.)

   Hint: $\frac{\text{ml } O_2}{\text{min}} \times \frac{.005 \text{ kcal}}{\text{ml } O_2} = \frac{\text{kcal}}{\text{min}}$
12. Given the $\dot{V}O_2$ in the units ml O_2/kg/min, determine the METs performed by a cycle rider using the O_2 consumption values given below. Remember to always write out the units. This way you are sure to avoid confusion.
   (a) 24.5 ml O_2/kg/min
   (b) 36 ml O_2/kg/min
   (c) 66.5 ml O_2/kg/min

Chapter 3 Answers to Practice Problems

1. 100 yd to ft $\quad 100 \cancel{\text{yd}} \times \frac{3 \text{ ft}}{1 \cancel{\text{yd}}} = 300 \text{ ft}$
2. 300 ft to in $\quad 300 \cancel{\text{ft}} \times \frac{12 \text{ in}}{1 \cancel{\text{ft}}} = 3{,}600 \text{ in}$
3. 3,600 in to cm $\quad 3{,}600 \cancel{\text{in}} \times \frac{2.54 \text{ cm}}{1 \cancel{\text{in}}} = 9{,}144 \text{ cm}$
4. 9,144 cm to m $\quad 9{,}144 \cancel{\text{cm}} \times \frac{1 \text{ m}}{100 \cancel{\text{cm}}} = 91.44 \text{ m}$
5. 5 miles to km $\quad 5 \cancel{\text{miles}} \times \frac{1 \text{ km}}{.62 \cancel{\text{miles}}} = 8.1 \text{ km}$

Another conversion factor can also be used to convert miles to km.

$$5 \text{ miles} \times \frac{1.62 \text{ km}}{1 \text{ mile}} = 8.1 \text{ km}$$

6. $\dfrac{1 \text{ mile}}{25 \text{ min}}$ to mph

$$\frac{1 \text{ mile}}{25 \text{ min}} \times \frac{60 \text{ min}}{1 \text{ hr}} = \frac{2.4 \text{ mile}}{\text{hr}} \text{ or } 2.4 \text{ mph}$$

7. 2.4 mph to m/min $\quad 2.4 \text{ mph} \times \dfrac{26.8 \text{ m/min}}{1 \text{ mph}} = 64.32 \text{ m/min}$

8. Converting mph to the unit m/min
   (a) 83.08 m/min
   (b) 99.16 m/min
   (c) 201 m/min

9. (a) $57 \text{ m/min} \times \dfrac{1 \text{ mph}}{26.8 \text{ m/min}} = 2.13$ mph walking
   (b) 2.5 mph walking
   (c) 5.5 mph running

10. Determine kcal/min from relative $\dot{V}O_2$.
   (a) $\dfrac{20 \text{ ml } O_2}{\text{kg/min}} \times 80 \text{ kg} \times \dfrac{.005 \text{ kcal}}{\text{ml } O_2} = \dfrac{8 \text{ kcal}}{\text{min}}$
   (b) $12.8 \dfrac{\text{kcal}}{\text{min}}$

11. Determine kcal/min from absolute $\dot{V}O_2$.
   (a) $9.6 \dfrac{\text{kcal}}{\text{min}}$
   (b) $11 \dfrac{\text{kcal}}{\text{min}}$
   (c) $30.4 \dfrac{\text{kcal}}{\text{min}}$

12. Determine MET levels.
   (a) $24.5 \text{ ml } O_2\text{/kg/min} \times \dfrac{1 \text{ MET}}{3.5 \text{ ml } O_2\text{/kg/min}} = 7 \text{ METs}$
   (b) $36 \text{ ml } O_2\text{/kg/min} \times \dfrac{1 \text{ MET}}{3.5 \text{ ml } O_2\text{/kg/min}} = 10.29 \text{ METs}$
   (c) 19 MET (an Olympic marathon runner)

4 Cardiovascular Dynamics and Calculations

Major Concepts

Cardiac output equation, $\dot{Q} = HR \times SV$

Arteriovenous oxygen difference, a-$\bar{v}$ O_2 diff

Fick equation, $\dot{V}O_2 = \dot{Q} \times$ a-$\bar{v}$ O_2 diff

Oxygen pulse, O_2 pulse $= \dot{V}O_2/HR$

Double product (rate-pressure product), $DP = \dfrac{HR \times SBP}{100}$

Pulse pressure, pulse pressure $= SBP - DBP$

Mean arterial pressure, $MAP = \dfrac{SBP - DBP}{3} + DBP$

As you progress through this chapter you will gain an understanding of the relationships between SV, HR, $\dot{Q}$, a-$\bar{v}$ O_2 diff, $\dot{V}O_2$, EDV, ESV, and EF. This will prepare you for the mathematics and other physiological concepts discussed in the following chapters.

In this chapter we will consider the mathematics that deal with the amount of blood the heart pumps per beat and the general and specific changes that occur in the vascular system as someone goes from rest to exercise. It is assumed that the reader has an understanding of the anatomy of the heart and lungs and general knowledge of cardiovascular physiology.

Before discussing the mathematics that deal with the physiology of the heart and vascular system it will be useful to identify the components and terminology included in the Fick equation and other related concepts.

Fick Equation Terminology

oxygen uptake ($\dot{V}O_2$ or VO_2)—The volume of oxygen used by muscle and other body tissues. These values can be expressed as:

$\dot{V}O_2$ = ml O_2/kg/min (relative to body weight) or
$\dot{V}O_2$ = ml O_2/min (absolute) or
VO_2 = L O_2 (total over a period of time)

The dot above the *V* ($\dot{V}O_2$) means *per minute.* In certain situations the term VO_2 is written without a dot over the *V*. This means oxygen consumed over a period of time, such as 5 or 10 min of rest or exercise.

cardiac output ($\dot{Q}$)—The volume of blood pumped out of the left ventricle each minute (ml blood/min). The dot above the *Q* ($\dot{Q}$) means *per minute.*

arteriovenous oxygen difference (a-$\bar{v}$ O_2 diff)—The difference in oxygen content between the arterial blood and the mixed venous blood. The units for this value are ml O_2/100 ml blood. The small dash above the *v* in the term a-$\bar{v}$ O_2 diff indicates average mixed venous O_2 content. As a subject progresses from rest to exercise, more oxygen is extracted out of the arterial blood by working muscle, leaving less oxygen in the venous blood. The more O_2 extracted at the capillary bed level in the muscles and other tissues, the less O_2 will be left in the venous blood (Adamovich, 1984; Fox, Bowers, & Foss, 1988). In other words, an increase in exercise intensity equals a decrease in venous O_2 content.

stroke volume (SV)—The volume of blood pumped out of the left ventricle, per beat, expressed as ml blood/bt. In a normal healthy heart, the right and left ventricles pump the same volume of blood each beat. The normal range of SV at rest is 70–90 ml blood/bt.

heart rate (HR)—The number of ventricular contractions per minute, expressed as bt/min or bpm.

end diastolic volume (EDV)—Milliliters of blood filling the left ventricle at the end of the each diastolic filling (rest) phase. Normal range at rest is 110–120 ml blood/bt.

ejection fraction (EF)—The fraction (expressed as a percentage) of the EDV of blood that is ejected from the left ventricle during systole. A small portion of blood remains in the left ventricle after each contraction. Ejection fraction is the percentage of blood pumped out each beat. Normal range at rest is 54–64%.

end systolic volume (ESV)—Milliliters of blood remaining in the left ventricle after each systolic pump (beat) phase. Normal range at rest is 40–50 ml blood/bt.

oxygen pulse (O_2 pulse)—$\dot{V}O_2$/HR, which is milliliters of O_2 consumed by the body per heartbeat, expressed as ml O_2/bt. Normal range at rest is 4–5 ml O_2/bt.

cardiac reserve—The ability of cardiac output ($\dot{Q}$) to increase from rest to exercise in order to meet oxygen and blood flow demands. By looking at the equation for cardiac output ($\dot{Q}$ = SV × HR), you will notice that *cardiac reserve* is directly influenced by HR and SV. Both HR and SV increase with exercise intensity, resulting in increased cardiac output.

The Fick Equation

The Fick equation describes the relationships among cardiac output, oxygen consumption, and arteriovenous oxygen difference. The basic Fick equation is written

$$\dot{V}O_2 = \dot{Q} \times \text{a-}\bar{v}\ O_2 \text{ diff}$$

Cardiac output ($\dot{Q}$) is the product of heart rate and stroke volume. Stroke volume, in turn, is the product of end diastolic volume and ejection fraction (see the sidebar on the facing page to review terminology). Knowing these facts, you can manipulate the Fick equation in several ways. Each of the following equations is a different way of writing the Fick equation:

$$\dot{V}O_2 = \dot{Q} \times \text{a-}\bar{v}\ O_2 \text{ diff}$$
$$\dot{V}O_2 = SV \times HR \times \text{a-}\bar{v}\ O_2 \text{ diff}$$
$$\dot{V}O_2 = EDV \times EF \times HR \times \text{a-}\bar{v}\ O_2 \text{ diff}$$
$$\frac{\dot{V}O_2}{\dot{Q}} = \text{a-}\bar{v}\ O_2 \text{ diff}$$
$$\dot{Q} = \frac{\dot{V}O_2}{\text{a-}\bar{v}\ O_2 \text{ diff}}$$

Examples 4A through 4G provide practice with using the Fick equation to find different values.

Example 4A

Determine cardiac output ($\dot{Q}$). Mr. Smith is a 30-year-old male. His heart rate (HR) is 60 bt/min and stroke volume (SV) is 70 ml blood/bt. Find $\dot{Q}$.

Step 1: Set up the equation.

$$HR \times SV = \dot{Q}$$

Step 2: Fill in known values.

$$\frac{60 \cancel{\text{bt}}}{\text{min}} \times \frac{70 \text{ ml blood}}{\cancel{\text{bt}}} = \dot{Q}$$

Step 3: Calculate.

$$\frac{4{,}200 \text{ ml blood}}{\text{min}} = \dot{Q} \text{ or } \frac{4.20 \text{ L blood}}{\text{min}}$$

With an HR of 60 bt/min and an SV of 70 ml blood/bt, this subject must be at rest. A $\dot{Q}$ of 4,200 ml blood/min is a resting value (see Table 4.1).

Example 4B

Find absolute and relative $\dot{V}O_2$. Mr. Smith, from Example 4A, has an a-$\bar{v}$ O_2 diff of 7 ml O_2/100 ml blood. You found his cardiac output is 4,200 ml blood/min. You have been asked to calculate his absolute oxygen consumption and his oxygen consumption relative to body weight. Mr. Smith weighs 70 kg.

Step 1: Write out the Fick equation.

$$\text{a-}\bar{v}\ O_2 \text{ diff} \times \dot{Q} = \dot{V}O_2$$

Table 4.1 Fick Components and Average Values

	Healthy (30 year old)		*Post MI (65 year old)
	Untrained	**Trained**	**Heart disease**
Heart rate (bt/min)			
Rest	72	50	70
Maximal effort	190	196	126
Stroke volume (ml blood/bt)			
Rest	70	110	**60
Maximal effort	150	180	**80
Cardiac output (ml blood/min)			
Rest	5,000	5,000	4,200
Maximal effort	20,000	29,000	10,000
Ejection fraction (%)			
Rest	58	60	**40
Maximal effort	80	82	**50
a-$\bar{v}$ O_2 diff (ml O_2/100 ml blood)			
Rest	6	6	6
Maximal effort	14	17	10
End diastolic volume (ml blood/bt)			
Rest	120	185	150
Maximal effort	180	225	160
End systolic volume (ml/blood/bt)			
Rest	50	75	90
Maximal effort	30	45	80
Oxygen pulse (ml O_2/bt)			
Rest	4.5	6	3.6
Maximal effort	15	30	8
Oxygen consumption, $\dot{V}O_2$ (ml O_2/min, absolute)			
Rest	280	300	250
Maximal effort	3,000	5,000	2,000
Oxygen consumption, $\dot{V}O_2$ (ml O_2/kg/min, relative for an 80-kg subject)			
Rest	3.5 (1 MET)	3.75	3.1
Maximal effort	37.5	62.5	25

Note. The units included within this table are bt/min, ml blood/bt, ml blood/min, %, ml O_2/100 ml blood, ml O_2/bt, and ml O_2/min.
* Post MI = after a myocardial infarction (heart attack).
** A severe MI may damage (weaken) the left ventricle enough so that EF and SV actually decrease with exercise.

Step 2: Enter the given values into the equation. Cancel the appropriate units and perform the math.

$$\frac{7\text{ ml }O_2}{100\text{ }\cancel{\text{ml blood}}} \times \frac{4{,}200\text{ }\cancel{\text{ml blood}}}{\text{min}} = \dot{V}O_2$$

$$\frac{294\text{ ml }O_2}{\text{min}} = \dot{V}O_2\text{ (absolute)}$$

Step 3: Divide the absolute $\dot{V}O_2$ by 70 kg to get the relative $\dot{V}O_2$.

$$\frac{294\text{ ml }O_2/\text{min}}{70\text{ kg}} = 4.2\text{ ml }O_2/\text{kg/min} = \dot{V}O_2\text{ (relative to wt)}$$

An absolute $\dot{V}O_2$ is the total value of oxygen uptake per minute. The relative $\dot{V}O_2$ value, on the other hand, is the oxygen uptake value per minute considering (relative to) the subject's body weight in kilograms.

Notice how conveniently the units cancel in examples 4A and 4B, confirming that you have the correct units for the answer. This will be very useful for identifying correct multiple choice answers on an exam.

Determining a-$\bar{v}$ O_2 diff

How was Mr. Smith's a-$\bar{v}$ O_2 diff determined? The determination of a-$\bar{v}$ O_2 diff is an invasive procedure requiring blood samples from the pulmonary and radial arteries. This is performed only in a hospital setting, not in a typical exercise physiology lab. The difference in the O_2 content between the arterial sample and the mixed venous sample represents the a-$\bar{v}$ O_2 diff (Guyton, 1991; McArdle et al., 1994).

An excellent discussion of a-$\bar{v}$ O_2 diff, $\dot{V}O_2$, SV, and $\dot{Q}$ can be found in the textbook *Principles of Exercise Testing and Interpretation* by Wasserman et al. (1987).

Example 4C

Find absolute $\dot{V}O_2$, $\dot{Q}$, and SV. A subject who weighs 72 kg is performing a graded exercise test (GXT) on a cycle ergometer, and the a-$\bar{v}$ O_2 diff and $\dot{V}O_2$ are recorded using an open-circuit spirometry/metabolic-cart system. See the textbook *Exercise Physiology* by McArdle et al. (1994, ch. 8) for a complete discussion of open-circuit spirometry.

Given the following measured values, find absolute $\dot{V}O_2$, $\dot{Q}$, and SV.

$$\dot{V}O_2 = 40\text{ ml }O_2/\text{kg/min}$$

$$\text{a-}\bar{v}\text{ }O_2\text{ diff} = \frac{14\text{ ml }O_2}{100\text{ ml blood}}$$

$$\text{HR} = \frac{150\text{ bt}}{\text{min}}$$

Step 1: Determine absolute $\dot{V}O_2$.

$$\frac{40\text{ ml }O_2}{\text{kg/min}} \times 72\text{ kg} = \frac{2{,}880\text{ ml }O_2}{\text{min}}$$

Step 2: Determine $\dot{Q}$.

$$\frac{\dot{V}O_2}{\text{a-}\bar{v}\ O_2\ \text{diff}} = \dot{Q}$$

$$\frac{\frac{2{,}880\ \text{ml}\ O_2}{\text{min}}}{\frac{14\ \text{ml}\ O_2}{100\ \text{ml blood}}} = \dot{Q}$$

Step 3: Invert the denominator, cancel, and multiply.

$$\frac{2{,}880\ \cancel{\text{ml}\ O_2}}{\text{min}} \times \frac{100\ \text{ml blood}}{14\ \cancel{\text{ml}\ O_2}} = \dot{Q}$$

$$\frac{20{,}571\ \text{ml blood}}{\text{min}} = \dot{Q} \text{ or } \frac{20.57\ \text{L blood}}{\text{min}}$$

Step 4: Determine SV. Rearrange the equation to solve for SV.

$$\dot{Q} = SV \times HR$$

$$\frac{\dot{Q}}{HR} = SV$$

$$\frac{\frac{20{,}571\ \text{ml blood}}{\text{min}}}{\frac{150\ \text{bt}}{\text{min}}} = SV$$

Step 5: Invert the 150 bt/min, cancel, and multiply.

$$\frac{20{,}571\ \text{ml blood}}{\cancel{\text{min}}} \times \frac{\cancel{\text{min}}}{150\ \text{bt}} = SV$$

$$\frac{137.14\ \text{ml blood}}{\text{bt}} = SV$$

Example 4D

Find absolute and relative $\dot{V}O_2$. You are working with Barbara, who is performing a GXT on a stationary cycle. During the test Barbara begins to exhibit indicators that she is at her anaerobic or lactate threshold. At this point in her test Barbara's HR is 140 bt/min, her SV is 120 ml blood/bt, and she has an a-$\bar{v}$ O_2 diff of 13 ml O_2/100 ml blood. We are interested in determining absolute and relative oxygen uptake. Barbara weighs 72 kg.

Step 1: Write the Fick equation.

$$\dot{V}O_2 = HR \times SV \times \text{a-}\bar{v}\ O_2\ \text{diff}$$

Step 2: Enter the values, cancel the units, and perform the math.

$$\dot{V}O_2 = \frac{140 \cancel{\text{bt}}}{\text{min}} \times \frac{120 \cancel{\text{ml blood}}}{\cancel{\text{bt}}} \times \frac{13 \text{ ml } O_2}{100 \cancel{\text{ml blood}}}$$

$$\dot{V}O_2 = \frac{2{,}184 \text{ ml } O_2}{\text{min}} \quad (\text{absolute } \dot{V}O_2)$$

Step 3: Divide the absolute $\dot{V}O_2$ by Barbara's weight.

$$\dot{V}O_2 = \frac{2{,}184 \text{ ml } O_2/\text{min}}{72 \text{ kg}} = 30.33 \text{ ml } O_2/\text{kg}/\text{min} \quad (\text{relative } \dot{V}O_2)$$

Example 4E

Find SV. A weekend cyclist ended his GXT on a cycle ergometer at 6 min. When the test was stopped, the cyclist's HR was 150 bpm, his $\dot{V}O_2$ was 3,060 ml O_2/min, and he had an a-$\bar{v}$ O_2 diff of 17 ml O_2/100 ml blood. Find his stroke volume.

Step 1: Invert the denominator, cancel the units, and multiply.

$$\frac{\dot{V}O_2}{\text{a-}\bar{v}\ O_2 \text{ diff}} = \frac{\dfrac{3{,}060 \text{ ml } O_2}{\text{min}}}{\dfrac{17 \text{ ml } O_2}{100 \text{ ml blood}}} = \dot{Q}$$

$$\frac{3{,}060 \cancel{\text{ml } O_2}}{\text{min}} \times \frac{100 \text{ ml blood}}{17 \cancel{\text{ml } O_2}} = \dot{Q}$$

$$\frac{18{,}000 \text{ ml blood}}{\text{min}} = \dot{Q} \text{ or } \frac{18 \text{ L blood}}{\text{min}}$$

Step 2: Insert $\dot{Q}$ into the equation: $\dot{Q}/\text{HR} = \text{SV}$

$$\frac{\dot{Q}}{\text{HR}} = \frac{\dfrac{18{,}000 \text{ ml blood}}{\text{min}}}{\dfrac{150 \text{ bt}}{\text{min}}} = \text{SV}$$

Step 3: Invert the denominator, cancel, and multiply.

$$\frac{18{,}000 \text{ ml blood}}{\text{min}} \times \frac{\text{min}}{150 \text{ bt}} = \text{SV}$$

$$\frac{120 \text{ ml blood}}{\text{bt}} = \text{SV}$$

A cardiac output ($\dot{Q}$) of 18,000 ml blood/min and an SV of 120 ml blood/bt at the end of a cycle test that was stopped represents an untrained subject.

The Expanded Fick Equation and Related Math

Along with the discussion of SV, it is appropriate to consider the calculations for end diastolic volume (EDV), end systolic volume (ESV), and ejection fraction (EF) (Adamovich, 1984, p. 24; Guyton, 1991, p. 103). EDV is the volume of blood in the left ventricle at the end of the diastolic filling period. ESV is the volume of blood that remains in the left ventricle after each contraction. The EF is the percentage of blood pumped per heartbeat. EDV and EF can be added to the Fick equation as follows. Notice how the arrows link certain components.

$$\dot{V}O_2 = \dot{Q} \times a\text{–}\bar{v}\,O_2\,\text{diff}$$

$$\dot{V}O_2 = SV \times HR \times a\text{–}\bar{v}\,O_2\,\text{diff}$$

$$\dot{V}O_2 = EDV \times EF \times HR \times a\text{–}\bar{v}\,O_2\,\text{diff}$$

$$SV = EDV \times EF\text{, also written as } \frac{SV}{EDV} = EF$$

$$SV = EDV - ESV$$

Example 4F

Calculate SV and EF. If EDV is 120 ml blood/bt and ESV is 50 ml blood/bt, what are SV and EF? On the basis of these values, determine whether this subject is at rest or is exercising.

Step 1: Enter the values into the SV equation.

$$EDV - ESV = SV$$

$$\frac{120\text{ ml blood}}{\text{bt}} - \frac{50\text{ ml blood}}{\text{bt}} = SV$$

$$\frac{70\text{ ml blood}}{\text{bt}} = SV$$

Step 2: Use the SV from step 1 and determine EF.

$$\frac{SV}{EDV} = \frac{\frac{70\text{ ml blood}}{\text{bt}}}{\frac{120\text{ ml blood}}{\text{bt}}} = EF$$

$$\frac{70\,\cancel{\text{ml blood}}}{\cancel{\text{bt}}} \times \frac{\cancel{\text{bt}}}{120\,\cancel{\text{ml blood}}} = EF$$

$$.58\text{ or }58\% = EF$$

Approximately 58% of the EDV is pumped out during each beat.

Step 3: Determine SV using EDV and EF. Rearrange SV/EDV = EF so that it is written

$$EDV \times EF = SV$$

Then determine the SV:

$$\text{EDV} \times \text{EF} = \text{SV}$$

$$\frac{120 \text{ ml blood}}{\text{bt}} \times .58 = \text{SV}$$

$$\frac{70 \text{ ml blood}}{\text{bt}} = \text{SV}$$

By doing step 3, we have proven that the calculation in step 1 is correct. We obtained the same answer using different equations.

Are these resting or exercising values? In step 1, the SV value 70 ml blood/bt is a resting value for an untrained subject. An EF of 58% from step 2 is also a resting value, but could be a value for either a trained or an untrained subject. See Table 4.1.

Another arrangement of the Fick equation is provided in example 4G. Use your calculator to follow the math steps.

Example 4G

Find SV. You are given values of 60% for EF and 130 ml blood/bt for EDV. You will notice in this example that EF has a percentage for the unit and EDV has ml blood/bt as units. Thus, SV will have the units ml blood/bt.

Step 1: Write the equation.

$$\text{EDV} \times \text{EF} = \text{SV}$$

Step 2: Fill in the values and calculate.

$$\frac{130 \text{ ml blood}}{\text{bt}} \times .60 = \text{SV}$$

$$\frac{78 \text{ ml blood}}{\text{bt}} = \text{SV}$$

These values represent a subject at rest. At a resting HR of 70 bt/min, cardiac output ($\dot{Q}$) would be 5,460 ml blood/min.

$$\text{SV} \times \text{HR} = \dot{Q}$$

$$\frac{78 \text{ ml blood}}{\cancel{\text{bt}}} \times \frac{70 \cancel{\text{bt}}}{\text{min}} = \dot{Q}$$

$$\frac{5{,}460 \text{ ml blood}}{\text{min}} = \dot{Q}$$

Oxygen Pulse and Double Product

You will find within the discussion of oxygen pulse (O_2 pulse) and double product, and in the next section pulse pressure and mean arterial pressure (MAP), components that you are familiar with from the Fick equation. Knowledge of these measures will provide you with additional tools that are valuable for analysis of an exercise test and evaluation of progress after a period of exercise training.

Oxygen Pulse (O_2 Pulse)

Oxygen pulse is a value used to indicate the volume of oxygen consumed by muscle and other tissues per heartbeat. O_2 pulse is also an indication of the volume of O_2 added to the pulmonary blood flow per heartbeat. The unit for O_2 pulse is ml O_2/bt. There are three variations to the O_2 pulse equation:

1. $O_2 \text{ pulse} = \frac{\dot{V}O_2}{HR}$. If $\dot{V}O_2 = \dot{Q} \times \text{a-}\bar{v}\ O_2 \text{ diff}$, then

2. $O_2 \text{ pulse} = \frac{\dot{Q} \times \text{a-}\bar{v}\ O_2 \text{ diff}}{HR}$. If $\dot{Q} = SV \times HR$, then

   $O_2 \text{ pulse} = \frac{SV \times HR \times \text{a-}\bar{v}\ O_2 \text{ diff}}{HR}$.

   The HRs cancel each other out, leaving the following equation:

3. $O_2 \text{ pulse} = SV \times \text{a-}\bar{v}\ O_2 \text{ diff}$

Example 4H illustrates equation 3. Example 4I uses equation 1 to solve for O_2 pulse.

Example 4H

Find O_2 pulse. For a subject whose SV is 66.67 and a-v̄ O_2 diff is 6 before the start of an exercise test, calculate the O_2 pulse.

Step 1: Write out the equation that will accept the values you have been given.

$$O_2 \text{ pulse} = SV \times \text{a-}\bar{v}\ O_2 \text{ diff}$$

Step 2: Enter the values into the equation, cancel, and perform the math.

$$O_2 \text{ pulse} = \frac{66.67 \cancel{\text{ml blood}}}{\text{bt}} \times \frac{6 \text{ ml } O_2}{100 \cancel{\text{ml blood}}}$$

$$O_2 \text{ pulse} = \frac{4.00 \text{ ml } O_2}{\text{bt}}$$

The O_2 pulse equation in example 4I, which uses $\dot{V}O_2$ and HR, is the equation found most often in textbooks and on physiology exams.

Example 4I

Find O_2 pulse. Using these values (from the subject in Example 4H), calculate O_2 pulse:

$$\dot{V}O_2 = \frac{280 \text{ ml } O_2}{\text{min}}$$

$$HR = \frac{70 \text{ bt}}{\text{min}}$$

Step 1: Write the equation that will accept the values you've been given.

$$O_2 \text{ pulse} = \frac{\dot{V}O_2}{HR}$$

Step 2: Enter the values into the equation. Invert the 70 bt/min, cancel, and perform the math.

$$O_2 \text{ pulse} = \frac{\frac{280 \text{ ml } O_2}{\text{min}}}{\frac{70 \text{ bt}}{\text{min}}}$$

$$O_2 \text{ pulse} = \frac{280 \text{ ml } O_2}{\cancel{\text{min}}} \times \frac{\cancel{\text{min}}}{70 \text{ bt}}$$

$$O_2 \text{ pulse} = \frac{4.00 \text{ ml } O_2}{\text{bt}}$$

Although different values were used in examples 4H and 4I, both examples have the same answer because the values were recorded from the same subject at the same time.

For more information about O_2 pulse, see Fox et al. (1988), Langler (1971), and Vander, Sherman, and Luciano (1975).

Double Product (Rate-Pressure Product)

The double product, also referred to as the rate-pressure product, is used as an indication of myocardial oxygen demand ($M\dot{V}O_2$). (See ACSM, 1988; Guyton, 1991; Langler, 1971). It is calculated from heart rate and the systolic blood pressure, one of the two components of blood pressure. (Systolic blood pressure [SBP] represents arterial pressure during the ventricle contraction [pumping] phase of the cardiac cycle, also referred to as systole. The diastolic blood pressure [DBP] represents arterial pressure during the cardiac phase of ventricle filling, also referred to as diastole.)

$$\text{Double product } (M\dot{V}O_2) = \frac{HR \times SBP}{100}$$

where HR = heart rate
SBP = systolic blood pressure

The term double product is used because two values are multiplied together to yield a product.

During increasing intensity of exercise, cardiac muscle increases its demands for oxygen due to a faster HR and more forceful contractions. In a normal healthy heart, $M\dot{V}O_2$ (myocardial O_2 demand) increases during exercise, as do blood flow and O_2 transport to the heart muscle. In this normal situation, oxygen supply is the same as oxygen demand.

On the other hand, in a patient with ischemic heart disease, at a given level of effort O_2 supply lags somewhat behind the demand for O_2. The result is *myocardial ischemia*. Myocardial ischemia usually produces anginal symptoms and ST wave

ECG changes. Anginal symptoms can occur in a variety of locations, such as the chest, jaw, shoulders, center of back, and arms.

The level of exercise intensity that produces myocardial ischemia, called the *ischemic threshold*, can be identified in an individual patient by noting the combination of HR and SBP. The double product can be used to maintain a cardiac patient's exercise intensity below the ischemic threshold. Example 4J illustrates the math for determining double product, that is, estimating the $M\dot{V}O_2$, at the end of a GXT.

Calculating the Double Product

Example 4J

A patient develops anginal pain during a GXT at an HR of 120 bt/min and an SBP of 180 mmHg. Find the double product.

Step 1: Write the equation.

$$\text{Double product} = \frac{\text{HR} \times \text{SBP}}{100}$$

Step 2: Insert the values and do the math.

$$\text{Double product} = \frac{\frac{120\ \cancel{\text{bt}}}{\text{min}} \times \frac{180\ \text{mmHg}}{\cancel{\text{bt}}}}{100} = 216\ \text{mmHg/min}$$

The value 216 mmHg/min, an index of $M\dot{V}O_2$, represents this patient's ischemic threshold. The recommendation for this patient would be to exercise below an intensity that produces a double product of 216. The double product number is most often written without the units.

Pulse Pressure and Mean Arterial Pressure

We turn now to two important issues that the exercise professional should not fail to analyze. Pulse pressure and mean arterial pressure are important aspects of the physiology related to blood pressure.

Pulse Pressure

Pulse pressure (Guyton, 1991; Langler, 1971) is defined as the difference between SBP and DBP. Written mathematically, pulse pressure = SBP − DBP. The word *pulse* in the term pulse pressure means "pulsating." The pulsating pressure between the diastolic and systolic alternates during each heartbeat. The pressure pulsates between the diastolic pressure and the systolic pressure during one heartbeat cycle. The pulse pressure, then, is the range between the upper and lower pressures.

Two factors affect pulse pressure: stroke volume (SV) and resistance to blood flow in the arterial system (peripheral resistance). When arteries throughout the body become hardened with arteriosclerosis, blood flow during rest and exercise becomes hampered by the peripheral resistance of the plaque-constricted artery lumen. This situation widens (increases) the pulse pressure, especially during exercise, as you will see when doing the practice problems.

Example 4K

Find pulse pressure. Use the values from Example 4J and a DBP of 94 mmHg to find the pulse pressure at the $M\dot{V}O_2$ ischemic threshold.

Step 1: Write the equation.

SBP − DBP = pulse pressure

Step 2: Fill in the values and do the math.

180 mmHg − 94 mmHg = pulse pressure

86 mmHg = pulse pressure

The value 86 mmHg is the pulsating range between the SBP and the DBP.

Mean Arterial Pressure

The mean (average) arterial pressure (MAP) is a measure of the average pressure in the vascular system. MAP is less than the average between systolic and diastolic pressure because the diastolic phase of the cardiac cycle is about one third longer than the systolic phase. Therefore,

$$\text{MAP} = \frac{\text{SBP} - \text{DBP}}{3} + \text{DBP}$$

For a healthy adult at rest with a blood pressure of 122/80 mmHg, the mean arterial pressure would be 94 mmHg: (122 − 80)/3 + 80 = 94 mmHg.

Chapter 4 Practice Problems

When calculating blood pressures and heart rate values, round off the numbers to the nearest whole number. Blood pressure numbers are traditionally recorded using even number values such as 140/76 rather than 139/77.

1. Given the following information, determine cardiac output ($\dot{Q}$).

	SV	HR	$\dot{Q}$
(a)	$\frac{65 \text{ ml blood}}{\text{bt}}$	$\frac{80 \text{ bt}}{\text{min}}$ =	
(b)	$\frac{110 \text{ ml blood}}{\text{bt}}$	$\frac{140 \text{ bt}}{\text{min}}$ =	

2. Write out the units for the following components of the Fick equation.

   Example: HR = 72 $\quad\quad$ $\text{HR} = 72 \frac{\text{bt}}{\text{min}}$

   (a) SV = 68

   (b) $\dot{Q}$ = 6,200

   (c) $\dot{Q}$ = 6.20

   (d) a-$\bar{v}$ O_2 diff = 6

   (e) HR = 84

   (f) EF = 68

(g) $\dot{V}O_2 = 4$

(h) $\dot{V}O_2 = 288 \frac{\quad}{min}$

(i) $\dot{V}O_2 = .4 \underline{\quad O_2}$

(j) SV = 108

(k) EDV $= 120 \frac{\quad}{bt}$

(l) ESV $= 60 \frac{\quad}{bt}$

3. Part A. The Fick equation. Draw in the arrows.

$$\dot{V}O_2 = \dot{Q} \times \text{a-}\bar{v}\ O_2 \text{ diff}$$

$$\dot{V}O_2 = SV \times HR \times \text{a-}\bar{v}\ O_2 \text{ diff}$$

$$\dot{V}O_2 = EDV \times EF \times HR \times \text{a-}\bar{v}\ O_2 \text{ diff}$$

Part B. In the following equations, fill in the blanks (?) with the correct component(s).

(a) $\dot{V}O_2 = ? \times \text{a-}\bar{v}\ O_2 \text{ diff}$

(b) $\frac{\dot{V}O_2}{\dot{Q}} = ?$

(c) $\dot{Q} = SV \times ?$

(d) $SV = EDV \times ?$

(e) $\frac{\dot{Q}}{SV} = ?$

(f) $\dot{V}O_2 = ? \times EF \times HR \times ?$

(g) $\frac{SV}{EDV} = ?$

(h) $\dot{Q} = \frac{?}{\text{a-}\bar{v}\ O_2 \text{ diff}}$

(i) $\dot{Q} = ? \times ?$

4. Determine HR, using the following information.

	$\dot{Q}$	SV
(a)	$\frac{4{,}800 \text{ ml blood}}{min}$	$\frac{80 \text{ ml blood}}{bt}$
(b)	$\frac{21{,}000 \text{ ml blood}}{min}$	$\frac{165 \text{ ml blood}}{bt}$

5. Given the following, determine the absolute $\dot{V}O_2$ values.
The units for each answer should be ml O_2/min.
Hint: Review the combinations in problem 3.

(a) $SV = \frac{120 \text{ ml blood}}{bt}$ $\quad HR = \frac{150 \text{ bt}}{min}$ $\quad \text{a-}\bar{v}\ O_2 \text{ diff} = \frac{17 \text{ ml } O_2}{100 \text{ ml blood}}$

(b) $\dot{Q} = \frac{18{,}000 \text{ ml blood}}{\text{min}}$ a-$\bar{v}$ O_2 diff $= \frac{17 \text{ ml } O_2}{100 \text{ ml blood}}$

(c) $HR = \frac{135 \text{ bt}}{\text{min}}$ $SV = \frac{128 \text{ ml blood}}{\text{bt}}$ a-$\bar{v}$ O_2 diff $= \frac{15 \text{ ml } O_2}{100 \text{ ml blood}}$

(d) $\dot{Q} = \frac{6{,}625 \text{ ml blood}}{\text{min}}$ a-$\bar{v}$ O_2 diff $= \frac{12 \text{ ml } O_2}{100 \text{ ml blood}}$

6. Determine a-$\bar{v}$ O_2 diff using the following information. These values were measured during an exercise test using a cycle ergometer. For each set of values, assess your answer to determine whether these values were measured just prior to starting the workload phase (resting) or during the exercise period.

	Arterial value	Mixed venous value
(a)	$\frac{18 \text{ ml } O_2}{100 \text{ ml blood}}$	$\frac{12 \text{ ml } O_2}{100 \text{ ml blood}}$
(b)	$\frac{19 \text{ ml } O_2}{100 \text{ ml blood}}$	$\frac{14 \text{ ml } O_2}{100 \text{ ml blood}}$
(c)	$\frac{19 \text{ ml } O_2}{100 \text{ ml blood}}$	$\frac{4 \text{ ml } O_2}{100 \text{ ml blood}}$

7. Given the following information, which of the values and units is correct for $\dot{Q}$?

Given: $\dot{V}O_2 = \frac{2{,}880 \text{ ml } O_2}{\text{min}}$

a-$\bar{v}$ O_2 diff $= \frac{14 \text{ ml } O_2}{100 \text{ ml blood}}$

(a) 2,062 ml O_2/bt
(b) 20,571 bt/min
(c) 20.57 L blood/min
(d) 403 ml/kg/min

8. Given the following information, determine SV and EF. The SV equation leads directly into the EF equation.

$EDV - ESV = SV$ and $\frac{SV}{EDV} = EF$

	End diastolic volume (EDV)	End systolic volume (ESV)
(a)	$\frac{120 \text{ ml blood}}{\text{bt}}$	$\frac{45 \text{ ml blood}}{\text{bt}}$
(b)	$\frac{116 \text{ ml blood}}{\text{bt}}$	$\frac{36 \text{ ml blood}}{\text{bt}}$
(c)	$\frac{118 \text{ ml blood}}{\text{bt}}$	$\frac{80 \text{ ml blood}}{\text{bt}}$
(d)	$\frac{114 \text{ ml blood}}{\text{bt}}$	$\frac{74 \text{ ml blood}}{\text{bt}}$

9. There are three basic equations for determining oxygen pulse. Complete the following three equations.

   (a) $O_2\ ? = \dfrac{?}{HR}$

   (b) $O_2 \text{ pulse} = \dfrac{\dot{Q} \times ?}{?}$

   (c) $O_2 \text{ pulse} = ? \times \text{a-}\bar{v}\ O_2 \text{ diff}$

10. Determine O_2 pulse for each of the following. Memory key: Resting $\dot{V}O_2$ is approximately 3.5 ml O_2/kg/min.

    (a) Is this subject at rest or performing strenuous exercise? What are your clues? Find O_2 pulse.

    $HR = \dfrac{186 \text{ bt}}{\text{min}}$ $\quad \dot{V}O_2 = \dfrac{2{,}825 \text{ ml } O_2}{\text{min}}$

    (b) This subject's true resting HR is 58 bt/min. The value 5 ml O_2/kg/min for $\dot{V}O_2$ is a clue that very light activity is being performed. Find O_2 pulse.

    $HR = \dfrac{72 \text{ bt}}{\text{min}}$ $\quad \dot{V}O_2 = \dfrac{5 \text{ ml } O_2}{\text{kg/min}}$ $\quad$ wt = 68 kg

    (c) $HR = \dfrac{110 \text{ bt}}{\text{min}}$ $\quad \dot{V}O_2 = 24 \text{ ml } O_2\text{/kg/min}$ $\quad$ wt = 92 kg

    (d) $HR = \dfrac{134 \text{ bt}}{\text{min}}$ $\quad \dot{V}O_2 = \dfrac{2{,}285 \text{ ml } O_2}{\text{min}}$

11. Determine double product ($M\dot{V}O_2$) at each stage of a cycle graded exercise test.

    Stages

    1. SBP = 130 HR = 80 DBP = 80
    2. SBP = 148 HR = 96 DBP = 90
    3. SBP = 180 HR = 140 DBP = 110

12. A patient with effort-induced angina has a double product ($M\dot{V}O_2$) threshold of 250. Which of the following combinations will produce angina with this patient?

	(bt/min)	(mmHg)
(a)	HR = 115	SBP = 220
(b)	HR = 120	SBP = 160
(c)	HR = 98	SBP = 210
(d)	HR = 180	SBP = 150

13. Determine pulse pressure for each of the following cases. All blood pressures are in the units mmHg. All heart rates are in the units bt/min.

    (a) SBP = 180 DBP = 90 HR = 180

    (b) DBP = 88 SBP = 164 HR = 165

14. Determine the mean arterial pressure (MAP) for each of the following cases. After you have double-checked your measurements, which of these people would you send directly to a doctor for further evaluation?

(a) SBP = 140 DBP = 90 (resting)

(b) DBP = 94 SBP = 164 (exercise)

(c) DBP = 86 SBP = 136 (exercise)

(d) SBP = 168 DBP = 70 (resting)

(e) DBP = 110 SBP = 220 (resting)

Chapter 4 Answers to Practice Problems

1. (a) $\dot{Q} = \frac{65 \text{ ml blood}}{\cancel{\text{bt}}} \times \frac{80 \cancel{\text{bt}}}{\text{min}}$

$\dot{Q} = \frac{5{,}200 \text{ ml blood}}{\text{min}}$ or $\frac{5.20 \text{ L blood}}{\text{min}}$

(b) $\frac{15{,}400 \text{ ml blood}}{\text{min}}$ or $\frac{15.40 \text{ L blood}}{\text{min}}$

2. (a) $SV = \frac{68 \text{ ml blood}}{\text{bt}}$

(b) $\dot{Q} = \frac{6{,}200 \text{ ml blood}}{\text{min}}$

(c) $\dot{Q} = \frac{6.20 \text{ L blood}}{\text{min}}$

(d) $\text{a-}\bar{\text{v}}\ O_2 \text{ diff} = \frac{6 \text{ ml } O_2}{100 \text{ ml blood}}$

(e) $HR = \frac{84 \text{ bt}}{\text{min}}$

(f) EF = 68%

(g) $\dot{V}O_2 = 4 \text{ ml } O_2/\text{kg/min}$

(h) $\dot{V}O_2 = \frac{288 \text{ ml } O_2}{\text{min}}$

(i) $\dot{V}O_2 = \frac{.4 \text{ L } O_2}{\text{min}}$

(j) $SV = \frac{108 \text{ ml blood}}{\text{bt}}$

(k) $EDV = \frac{120 \text{ ml blood}}{\text{bt}}$

(l) $ESV = \frac{60 \text{ ml blood}}{\text{bt}}$

3. Part A.

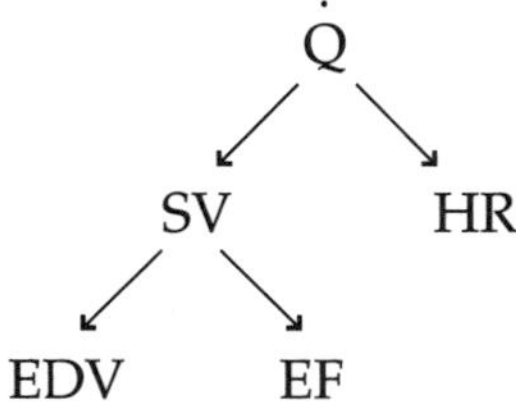

Part B.

(a) $\dot{Q}$

(b) a-$\bar{v}$ O_2 diff

(c) HR

(d) EF

(e) HR

(f) EDV, a-$\bar{v}$ O_2 diff

(g) EF

(h) $\dot{V}O_2$

(i) SV × HR

4. (a) $\frac{\dot{Q}}{SV} = HR$

$$\frac{4{,}800 \cancel{\text{ml blood}}}{\text{min}} \times \frac{\text{bt}}{80 \cancel{\text{ml blood}}} = \frac{60 \text{ bt}}{\text{min}} = \text{HR}$$

(b) 127 bt/min = HR

5. $\dot{V}O_2 = \dot{Q} \times$ a-$\bar{v}$ O_2 diff

or

$\dot{V}O_2 = HR \times SV \times$ a-$\bar{v}$ O_2 diff

(a) $\dot{V}O_2 = \frac{3{,}060 \text{ ml } O_2}{\text{min}}$ or $\frac{3.06 \text{ L } O_2}{\text{min}}$

(b) $\dot{V}O_2 = \frac{3{,}060 \text{ ml } O_2}{\text{min}}$

(c) $\dot{V}O_2 = \frac{2{,}592 \text{ ml } O_2}{\text{min}}$

(d) $\dot{V}O_2 = \frac{795 \text{ ml } O_2}{\text{min}}$

6. a-$\bar{v}$ O_2 diff

(a) 6 ml O_2/100 ml blood   resting value

(b) 5 ml O_2/100 ml blood   resting value

(c) 15 ml O_2/100 ml blood   high intensity exercise

7. (c) 20.57 L blood/min, $\frac{\dot{V}O_2}{\text{a-}\bar{v}\ O_2 \text{ diff}} = \dot{Q}$

or

20,571 ml blood/min

8. (a) $SV = \frac{75 \text{ ml blood}}{\text{bt}}$ EF = 62.5%

(b) $SV = \frac{80 \text{ ml blood}}{\text{bt}}$ EF = 69%

(c) $SV = \frac{38 \text{ ml blood}}{\text{bt}}$ $EF = 32\%$

(d) $SV = \frac{40 \text{ ml blood}}{\text{bt}}$ $EF = 35\%$

In (a) through (d), each EDV is near the normal range. In (c) and (d) the ESV values are 80 and 74, higher than in (a) and (b). In (c) and (d) less blood is ejected per beat, indicating left ventricle dysfunction. EF is very low in (c) and (d).

9. (a) $O_2 \text{ pulse} = \frac{\dot{V}O_2}{HR}$

(b) $O_2 \text{ pulse} = \frac{\dot{Q} \times \text{a-}\bar{v}\ O_2 \text{ diff}}{HR}$

(c) $O_2 \text{ pulse} = SV \times \text{a-}\bar{v}\ O_2 \text{ diff}$

10. (a) $O_2 \text{ pulse} = \frac{\dot{V}O_2}{HR}$

$O_2 \text{ pulse} = \frac{2{,}825 \text{ ml } O_2}{\text{min}} \times \frac{\text{min}}{186 \text{ bt}}$

$O_2 \text{ pulse} = \frac{15.19 \text{ ml } O_2}{\text{bt}}$

(b) $O_2 \text{ pulse} = 4.72 \frac{\text{ml } O_2}{\text{bt}}$

(c) $O_2 \text{ pulse} = 20.07 \frac{\text{ml } O_2}{\text{bt}}$

(d) $O_2 \text{ pulse} = 17.05 \frac{\text{ml } O_2}{\text{bt}}$

11. (1) $\frac{HR \times SBP}{100} = 104 = \text{double product}$

(2) Double product = 142 mmHg

(3) Double product = 252 mmHg = anginal threshold

12. (a) = Double product = 253 = angina

(d) = Double product = 270 = angina

13. (a) 90 = pulse pressure

(b) 76 = pulse pressure

14. (a) 107 = mean arterial pressure (MAP)

(b) 117 = MAP

(c) 103 = MAP

(d) 103 = MAP

(e) 147 = MAP

Subject (e) would be sent to his/her doctor as soon as possible.

5 Pulmonary Function Calculations

Major Concepts

Standardizing pulmonary air and gas values; ATPS, BTPS, and STPD corrections

Calculating minute ventilation ($\dot{V}E$)

Calculating dead space (DS)

Calculating alveolar ventilation ($\dot{V}A$)

Calculating "wasted ventilation" (DS/TV)

Calculating O_2 consumption using pulmonary values

Calculating CO_2 production using pulmonary values

Absolute and relative $\dot{V}O_2$

In this chapter we will examine the mathematics involving pulmonary ventilation (air) and gas (O_2 and CO_2) exchange. The physiology of pulmonary ventilation will be discussed only to the extent required to provide insight into the related mathematics. It is assumed the reader has an understanding of pulmonary anatomy and related physiology.

Standardizing Pulmonary Gas Values: ATPS, BTPS, and STPD Conversions

Before surveying the mathematics related to pulmonary values such as minute ventilation ($\dot{V}E$), alveolar ventilation ($\dot{V}A$), O_2 consumption, and CO_2 production,

Abbreviations and Terms in Chapter 5

ATPS—Ambient temperature and pressure saturated with water. These are testing-room conditions. Ambient = atmospheric.

STPD—Standard temperature and pressure under dry conditions. Standard temperature is 0 °C; standard pressure is 760 mmHg (barometric pressure). "Dry" means that the air or gas contains no water vapor.

BTPS—Body temperature and pressure, saturated with water. Body temperature is about 37 °C. Pressure is barometric pressure (PB), which is the atmospheric pressure read from a barometer within the testing area. Normal range of PB is 700 to 770 mmHg. Average for PB is about 760 mmHg. "Saturated" means that the air is saturated with water vapor.

$\dot{V}E$—Minute ventilation, the total volume of air that is exhaled in 1 min. $\dot{V}E$ is expressed as ml air/min = TV × *f*.

f—Frequency of breaths/min.

TV—Tidal volume, the volume of air exhaled in one breath. TV is expressed as ml air/breath.

VC—Vital capacity, the maximal volume of air forcefully expired after a maximal inspiration.

$\dot{V}A$—Alveolar ventilation, the volume of air that reaches the lung alveoli.

DS—Physiologic dead space; includes anatomical DS and alveolar DS, which is the volume of air that does not participate in gas exchange.

$\dot{V}O_2$—The volume and rate per minute at which oxygen is consumed by the body. $\dot{V}O_2$ is expressed as ml O_2/min, ml O_2/kg/min, or L O_2/min.

$\dot{V}CO_2$—The volume and rate per minute of carbon dioxide gas production. $\dot{V}CO_2$ is expressed as ml CO_2/min or L CO_2/min. This value is not, as a rule, expressed in the units ml CO_2/kg/min.

it is necessary to discuss the methods of standardizing these values (Fox et al., 1988; McArdle et al., 1994; Wasserman et al., 1987). Standardizing these volumes of air and gas (O_2 and CO_2) involves correcting them from ATPS to STPD, ATPS to BTPS, or BTPS to STPD.

Because gas volumes vary with pressure and temperature they must be standardized so valid comparisons can be made, just as, when determining a distance, all units of measure must be corrected to the same linear unit or standard.

Open-circuit spirometry measures the air and gas values during rest and exercise by collecting and analyzing a subject's expired air volumes. The valve at the mouthpiece separates inspired air from the expired air. The expired air volumes are measured through use of a flow meter to determine $\dot{V}E$. The percentages of oxygen (O_2) and carbon dioxide (CO_2) are measured by an electronic gas analyzer.

All three of the basic pulmonary values, $\dot{V}E$, $\dot{V}O_2$, and $\dot{V}CO_2$, are calculated from expired air. When a person breathes into the spirometer mouthpiece, valve, and tubing, the air coming from the lungs is at BTPS, which is at 37 °C and saturated with water vapor. As the air travels through the valve and tubing and toward the analyzer it begins to cool and equalize to ATPS conditions. This is due to Charles' law, which states that "as the temperature of a gas increases or decreases, its volume increases or decreases in direct proportion to the change in temperature."

You can use one of the following three equations to standardize the value. To correct volumes of air or gas at room (equipment) temperature (ATPS) back to volumes at body temperature (BTPS), use equation B. To correct from BTPS to STPD, use equation C. When an air or gas volume is already at ATPS, it can be corrected directly to STPD by using equation A.

A. $$V\ (STPD) = V\ (ATPS) \times \frac{K}{K + AT} \times \frac{P_B - P\ H_2O\ (room)}{SP_B}$$

B. $$V\ (BTPS) = V\ (ATPS) \times \frac{K + BT}{K + AT} \times \frac{P_B - P\ H_2O\ (room)}{P_B - P\ H_2O\ (lungs)}$$

Note: When correcting BTPS, BT (body temperature) is a factor in the equation.

C. $$V\ (STPD) = V\ (BTPS) \times \frac{K}{K + AT} \times \frac{P_B - P\ H_2O\ (lungs)}{SP_B}$$

V—Volume of any air or gas.

K—Kelvin temperature scale, K = 273 °. The Kelvin temperature scale is routinely used when air and gas volumes are studied; 0 °C = 273 °K. Why use the number 273 for Kelvin? When heated through 1 °C (0 °C to 1 °C), a volume of air or gas will expand 1/273 of its volume when the pressure remains unchanged.

BT—Body temperature = 37 °C = 98.6 °F. The Celsius scale is used in the correction equations.

AT—Atmospheric (ambient/room) temperature.

P_B—Barometric pressure in the testing room, expressed in mmHg.

SP_B—Standard barometric pressure at sea level, always equal to 760 mmHg.

P H_2O (room)—Water vapor pressure at room temperature.

P H_2O (lungs)—Water vapor pressure at lung temperature.

The *V* within each equation represents air ($\dot{V}E$, TV, or VC) or gas (O_2 or CO_2) volumes recorded per minute or over a period of several minutes. Air volumes can be corrected from ATPS to BTPS, then to STPD. But the best choice is to correct volumes of air at ATPS directly to STPD by using equation A.

Once $\dot{V}E$ (BTPS) is determined it can be recorded as $\dot{V}E$ (BTPS). The $\dot{V}E$ (BTPS) must then be corrected to STPD so that it can be used in $\dot{V}O_2$ and $\dot{V}CO_2$ math calculations. $\dot{V}O_2$ and $\dot{V}CO_2$ volumes are routinely expressed as the volumes they would occupy at STPD.

You will become more familiar with these concepts as you examine examples 5A and 5B and the practice problems at the end of this chapter.

Volume changes occur in three ways when these corrections are made:

1. ATPS to STPD—Volume decreases, as in example 5A (4 L becomes 3.55 L).
2. ATPS to BTPS—Volume increases, as in example 5B (9.5 L/min becomes 10.32 L/min).
3. BTPS to STPD—Volume decreases, as in practice problem 4.

Examine the standardization equations (Fox et al., 1988; McArdle et al., 1994; Wasserman et al., 1987) and work through the steps of the example problems to become familiar with standardizing air and gas volumes.

Example 5A

Correct a volume of collected expired CO_2 from ATPS to STPD. Expired VCO_2 (ATPS), 4 L, was collected under the following conditions (note that because this 4 L of VCO_2 is a total volume of gas collected over a period of several minutes there is no dot over the *V*):

$$\begin{aligned} K &= 273\ °K \\ AT &= 20\ °C \\ P_B &= 745 \text{ mmHg (from lab barometer)} \\ P\ H_2O \text{ (room)} &= 18 \text{ mmHg water vapor at } 20\ °C \text{ (from Table 5.1)} \\ SP_B &= 760 \text{ mmHg (standard barometric pressure at sea level)} \end{aligned}$$

What is the VCO_2 (STPD)?

Step 1: Write out equation A.

$$VCO_2\ (STPD) = VCO_2\ (ATPS) \times \frac{K}{K + AT} \times \frac{P_B - P\ H_2O\ (room)}{SP_B}$$

Table 5.1 Water Vapor Pressures at Different Temperatures

Temperatures		
°C	°F	P H_2O
20	68	18 mmHg
21	70	19
22	72	20
23	73	21
24	75	22
25	77	24
26	79	25
27	81	27
28	82	28
29	84	30
30	86	32
31	88	34
32	90	35
33	91	38
34	93	40
35	95	42
36	97	45
37	99	47
38	100	50
39	102	52
40	104	55

Note. This table is based upon Boyle's law, which states that as temperature increases or decreases so does the P H_2O (water vapor pressure).

Step 2: Insert the appropriate values and perform the math.

$$VCO_2 \text{ (STPD)} = 4 \text{ L (ATPS)} \times \frac{273\ °K}{273\ °K + 20\ °C} \times \frac{745 \text{ mmHg} - 18 \text{ mmHg}}{760 \text{ mmHg}}$$
$$VCO_2 \text{ (STPD)} = 4 \text{ L} \times .9285714 \times .9565789$$

Step 3: Round off the final answer.

$$VCO_2 \text{ (STPD)} = 3.5530072 = 3.55 \text{ L}$$

When correcting a volume from ATPS to STPD, the volume decreases. VCO_2 is always reported at STPD.

Example 5B

Correct a volume of air at ATPS to BTPS. The minute ventilation ($\dot{V}E$) for a subject at rest was 9.5 L of air per minute (ATPS). It was collected under the following conditions:

AT = 23 °C
P H_2O (room) = 21 mmHg at 23 °C
BT = 37 °C
P H_2O (lungs) = 47 mmHg at 37 °C body temp
PB = 752 mmHg from lab barometer

Correct this volume to BTPS.

Step 1: Write out equation B.

$$\dot{V}E \text{ (BTPS)} = \dot{V}E \text{ (ATPS)} \times \frac{K + BT}{K + AT} \times \frac{P_B - P\ H_2O \text{ (room)}}{P_B - P\ H_2O \text{ (lungs)}}$$

Step 2: Insert the values and perform the math.

$$\dot{V}E \text{ (BTPS)} = 9.5 \text{ L/min (ATPS)} \times \frac{273\ °K + 37\ °C}{273\ °K + 23\ °C} \times \frac{752 \text{ mmHg} - 21 \text{ mmHg}}{752 \text{ mmHg} - 47 \text{ mmHg}}$$
$$\dot{V}E \text{ (BTPS)} = 9.5 \text{ L/min} \times 1.0472972 \times 1.0368794$$
$$\dot{V}E \text{ (BTPS)} = 10.316248 = 10.32 \text{ L/min}$$

When the volume of air ($\dot{V}E$) at ATPS is corrected back to the conditions of the warmth of the lungs (BTPS), the volume expands.

With an understanding of standardized (corrected) air and gas volumes we can proceed to the use of $\dot{V}E$ (STPD), $\dot{V}O_2$ (STPD), and $\dot{V}CO_2$ (STPD) in metabolic math calculations. As you read through the rest of this chapter, assume that all air and gas values have already been corrected to STPD, unless otherwise specified. There are volume correction practice problems at the end of the chapter.

Minute Ventilation ($\dot{V}E$)

In breathing we inhale ($\dot{V}I$) and exhale ($\dot{V}E$) a volume of air each minute. (V = volume; I = inhale; E = exhale.)

Table 5.2 Average Ranges of Pulmonary Values for a Normal, Healthy Subject, Male or Female, Age 18–35, Moderate Level of Fitness

Variables	Rest	Maximal exercise
Tidal volume (TV) ml air/breath	400 to 500	2,500 to 3,000
Breathing frequency (*f*) breaths/min	10 to 20	40 to 45
Minute ventilation ($\dot{V}E$) ml air/min	4,000 to 10,000	100,000 to 135,000 (100 to 135 L air/min)
Alveolar ventilation ($\dot{V}A$) ml air/min	3,000 to 7,000	88,000 to 112,500 (88 to 112.5 L air/min)
Physiological dead space (DS) ml air/breath	100 to 150	300 to 500
Dead space/tidal volume ratio (DS/TV) %	25 to 30	12 to 16
Oxygen consumption ($\dot{V}O_2$) ml O_2/kg/min	3 to 4	30 to 50

Note. From *Resource Manual for Guidelines for Exercise Testing and Prescription* by ACSM, 1988, Philadelphia: Lea & Febiger.
The Physiological Basis of Physical Education and Athletics (pp. 208, 209, 212) by E. L. Fox, R. W. Bowers, and M. L. Foss, 1988, New York: Saunders.
Exercise Physiology: Energy, Nutrition and Human Performance (4th ed.) (ch. 21) by W. D. McArdle, W. D. Katch, and V. L. Katch, 1994, Philadelphia: Lea & Febiger.
Principles of Exercise Testing and Interpretation by K. Wasserman, J. E. Hansen, D. Y. Sue, and B. J. Whipp, 1987, Philadelphia: Lea & Febiger.

Minute ventilation ($\dot{V}E$), the total amount of air exhaled per minute (ml air/min), ranges from 4 L/min at rest to over 100 L/min during maximal exercise. Normal values for other pulmonary parameters are shown in Table 5.2.

$\dot{V}E$ (ml air/min) is the product of tidal volume and frequency.

$$\dot{V}E = TV \times f$$

Tidal volume (TV) is the volume of air exhaled per breath (ml air/breath); Frequency (*f*) is the number of breaths per minute (breaths/min).

Example 5C

Determine $\dot{V}E$. This subject is at rest. The ventilatory values have been determined through the use of a metabolic cart/open-circuit spirometry system. TV is 500 ml air/breath and *f* is 18 breaths/min. Assume that all values have already been corrected to STPD.

Step 1: Write out the $\dot{V}E$ equation.

$$\dot{V}E = TV \times f$$

Step 2: Enter the given values into the equation. Cancel the appropriate units and perform the math.

$$\dot{V}E = \frac{500 \text{ ml air}}{\cancel{\text{breath}}} \times \frac{18 \cancel{\text{ breaths}}}{\text{min}}$$

$$\dot{V}E = \frac{9{,}000 \text{ ml air}}{\text{min}} \text{ or } \frac{9 \text{ L air}}{\text{min}}$$

Keeping track of the units will ensure that there will be no confusion between ml air, ml blood, and ml O_2. There are mathematical practice problems at the end of the chapter that involve $\dot{V}E$ calculations.

Physiologic Dead Space (DS)

Physiologic dead space (DS) of the respiratory system consists of two components: anatomic and alveolar dead space. Physiologic dead space = anatomic dead space + alveolar dead space. Anatomic dead space consists of the volume of air in the mouth, nasal passages, trachea, bronchial tree, and other nondiffusible areas of the respiratory system. Alveolar dead space is the volume of air in the lungs contained in alveoli that are either damaged so they cannot hold air or that are poorly perfused with blood. In normal adults where all alveoli are functional, alveolar dead space is close to zero. However, in chronic obstructive lung disease (COPD) and other lung diseases, alveolar dead space can be considerable. Therefore, in normal individuals, physiologic dead space is equal or nearly equal, to the anatomical dead space. However, in lung disease patients, physiologic dead space can be as large as 1 to 2 L of air per breath because of the large number of damaged alveoli.

Anatomic dead space is difficult to measure precisely but can be estimated to an accuracy of plus or minus 10 ml of air based on body weight in pounds. For example, the estimated anatomic dead space for a 145-lb person would be about 145 ml air/breath. To determine alveolar dead space directly requires measurement of the partial pressure of O_2 and CO_2 in expired air and arterial blood. Equations requiring the measurement of the partial pressure of CO_2 in expired air and arterial blood, as well as tidal volume, are available to calculate physiologic dead space.

Alveolar Ventilation ($\dot{V}A$)

The volume of air that reaches the alveoli and participates in gas exchange is called alveolar ventilation ($\dot{V}A$) (ml air/min).

Two basic equations can be used to solve for $\dot{V}A$:

(A) $$\dot{V}A = \dot{V}E - (DS \times f)$$

and

(B) $$\dot{V}A = (TV - DS) \times f$$

Typical values for a subject at rest are TV of 500 ml/breath, DS of 150 ml/breath, and f of 12 breaths/min.

Using equation B from above,

$$\dot{V}A = \frac{(500 \text{ ml}}{\text{breath}} - \frac{150 \text{ ml})}{\text{breath}} \times \frac{12 \text{ breaths}}{\text{min}}$$

$$\dot{V}A = \frac{350 \text{ ml}}{\cancel{\text{breath}}} \times \frac{12 \cancel{\text{ breaths}}}{\text{min}}$$

$$\dot{V}A = 4{,}200 \text{ ml air/min}$$

Ratio of Dead Space to Tidal Volume (DS/TV)

The ratio (DS/TV) can provide information about the efficiency of blood circulation through the alveolar-capillary beds at the alveoli, which is considered the pulmonary circulation. This ratio also indicates the amount of ventilation per minute that is "wasted" and does not function as a transport for O_2 or CO_2. In practical terms it is a *functional advantage* for a subject to have as little "wasted" ventilation as possible, especially during exercise.

Examine the following examples that cover $\dot{V}E$, $\dot{V}A$, DS, and TV.

Example 5D

Determine alveolar ventilation ($\dot{V}A$). A subject had a resting $\dot{V}E$ of 10.4 L/min, or 10,400 ml; a TV of 866.67 ml air/breath; an f of 12 breaths/min; and physiologic DS of 200 ml air/breath. What is the $\dot{V}A$?

Step 1: Write out the $\dot{V}A$ equation.

$$\dot{V}A = \dot{V}E - (DS \times f)$$

Step 2: Insert the known values into the equation.

$$\dot{V}A = \frac{10{,}400 \text{ ml air}}{\text{min}} - \frac{(200 \text{ ml air}}{\cancel{\text{breath}}} \times \frac{12 \ \cancel{\text{breath}})}{\text{min}}$$

Step 3: Cancel the appropriate units and perform the math.

$$\dot{V}A = \frac{10{,}400 \text{ ml air}}{\text{min}} - \frac{2{,}400 \text{ ml air}}{\text{min}}$$

$$\dot{V}A = \frac{8{,}000 \text{ ml air}}{\text{min}} \text{ or } \frac{8.0 \text{ L air}}{\text{min}}$$

When $\dot{V}E$, $\dot{V}A$, and f are known, DS can be calculated by rearranging the equation from Example 5D. The following equation is illustrated in Example 5E.

$$DS = \frac{\dot{V}E - \dot{V}A}{f}$$

Example 5E

Determine physiological DS. Using the following resting values that have already been corrected to STPD, find DS.

$$\dot{V}E = \frac{7{,}200 \text{ ml air}}{\text{min}}$$

$$f = 15 \text{ breaths/min}$$

$$\dot{V}A = \frac{4{,}500 \text{ ml air}}{\text{min}}$$

$$TV = 480 \text{ ml air/breath}$$

Step 1: Write out the DS equation.

$$DS = \frac{\dot{V}E - \dot{V}A}{f}$$

$\dot{V}A$ can be subtracted from $\dot{V}E$ because the units are the same.

Step 2: Insert the known values into the DS equation.

$$DS = \frac{\frac{7{,}200 \text{ ml air}}{\text{min}} - \frac{4{,}500 \text{ ml air}}{\text{min}}}{\frac{15 \text{ breaths}}{\text{min}}}$$

Step 3: Invert the denominator, cancel the appropriate units, and perform the math.

$$DS = \frac{2{,}700 \text{ ml air}}{\cancel{\text{min}}} \times \frac{\cancel{\text{min}}}{15 \text{ breaths}}$$

$$DS = \frac{180 \text{ ml air}}{\text{breath}}$$

Example 5F

Determine $\dot{V}A$. Using the following values that have been corrected to STPD, find $\dot{V}A$.

$$TV = \frac{600 \text{ ml air}}{\text{breath}}$$

$$DS = \frac{170 \text{ ml air}}{\text{breath}}$$

$$f = \frac{14 \text{ breaths}}{\text{min}}$$

Step 1: Write out the equation that fits the given values.

$$\dot{V}A = (TV - DS) \times f$$

Step 2: Insert the known values.

$$\dot{V}A = \frac{(600 \text{ ml air}}{\text{breath}} - \frac{170 \text{ ml air})}{\text{breath}} \times \frac{14 \text{ breaths}}{\text{min}}$$

Step 3: Perform the appropriate math sequence.

$$\dot{V}A = \frac{430 \text{ ml air}}{\cancel{\text{breath}}} \times \frac{14 \cancel{\text{breaths}}}{\text{min}}$$

$$\dot{V}A = \frac{6{,}020 \text{ ml air}}{\text{min}}$$

Calculating $\dot{V}O_2$ and $\dot{V}CO_2$ Using Pulmonary Values

Oxygen uptake ($\dot{V}O_2$) reflects total metabolic energy production. Resting $\dot{V}O_2$ values average between 200 and 350 ml O_2/min. At maximal exercise a well trained athlete can consume as much as 6,000 ml O_2/min. Measurement of O_2 consumption ($\dot{V}O_2$) as well as CO_2 production ($\dot{V}CO_2$) are routinely recorded during each stage of a GXT.

$\dot{V}O_2$ and $\dot{V}CO_2$ can be determined on the basis of cardiovascular or pulmonary values. In chapter 4, the cardiovascular values of cardiac output ($\dot{Q}$) and a-$\bar{v}$ O_2 difference were used to calculate $\dot{V}O_2$ with the Fick equation. Collecting these values requires the use of invasive techniques. On the other hand, pulmonary values, such as the amount of O_2 consumed and the amount of CO_2 produced, can be gathered noninvasively by using a mouthpiece/valve/air-flow meter system with open-circuit spirometry equipment.

Fractional Components of Oxygen and Carbon Dioxide

The fractional components (the percentages of O_2 and CO_2) in expired air must be measured to calculate $\dot{V}O_2$ and $\dot{V}CO_2$. It is important to remember that inspired air contains 20.93% oxygen, 0.03% carbon dioxide, and the remainder, 79.04%, is mostly nitrogen.

Calculating Oxygen Consumption ($\dot{V}O_2$) and Carbon Dioxide Production ($\dot{V}CO_2$)

To calculate $\dot{V}O_2$ (the amount of oxygen consumed per minute) we need to know the amount of oxygen inhaled per minute, which is the volume of air inhaled times the fraction of air that is oxygen ($\dot{V}I \times FIO_2$), and the amount of oxygen exhaled per minute ($\dot{V}E \times FEO_2$). Therefore,

$$\dot{V}O_2 = (\dot{V}I \times FIO_2) - (\dot{V}E \times FEO_2) \quad (1)$$

FIO_2 will always be greater than FEO_2 because the body uses oxygen to fuel metabolic processes.

Carbon dioxide production ($\dot{V}CO_2$) can be calculated in an analogous manner. However, in this case the amount of CO_2 in expired air will always be greater than the amount in inspired air because CO_2 is a by-product of metabolic processes. Therefore,

$$\dot{V}CO_2 = (\dot{V}E \times FECO_2) - (\dot{V}I \times FICO_2) \quad (2)$$

Alternate $\dot{V}O_2$ & $\dot{V}CO_2$ Equations

If the volume of expired air ($\dot{V}E$) is equal to the volume of inspired air ($\dot{V}I$), then the equations for $\dot{V}O_2$ and $\dot{V}CO_2$ can be simplified:

$$\dot{V}O_2 = \dot{V}E\,(FIO_2 - FEO_2)$$

and

$$\dot{V}CO_2 = \dot{V}E\,(FECO_2 - FICO_2)$$

These alternate equations cannot be used when $\dot{V}E$ does not equal $\dot{V}I$, as occurs when $\dot{V}O_2$ is greater than $\dot{V}CO_2$ or vice versa, as is often the case during exercise. These equations are therefore appropriate only when the respiratory exchange rate (R) = $\dot{V}CO_2/\dot{V}O_2$ is equal to 1.

In practice, most laboratory systems do not measure $\dot{V}I$ but measure only $\dot{V}E$. Therefore, to determine $\dot{V}O_2$, $\dot{V}I$ must be calculated using the Haldane correction equations, which are based on the concept that nitrogen is neither produced nor consumed during metabolism.

$$\dot{V}I = \frac{\dot{V}E \text{ (measured)} \times FEN_2 \text{ (calculated)}}{FIN_2 \text{ (constant) } 79.04\%}$$

where

$\dot{V}E$ = measured with spirometer, etc., and

$FEN_2 = 1 - FEO_2 - FECO_2$ (both FEO_2 and $FECO_2$ are measured by gas analyzer)

If $\dot{V}I$ (volume of air inhaled) is measured, $\dot{V}E$ can be calculated from:

$$\dot{V}E = \frac{\dot{V}I \times FIN_2}{FEN_2}$$

Example 5G

Determine $\dot{V}O_2$, $\dot{V}CO_2$, METs, and R. Mary-Jean, who weighs 65 kg, is engaged in submaximal exercise on a treadmill at 3.3 mph on a 15% grade. The following data were collected:

$\dot{V}E$ (STPD) = 72 L air/min
FIO_2 = .2093 (room air) − given
$FICO_2$ = .0003 (room air) − given
FEO_2 = .1595 (from O_2 analyzer)
$FECO_2$ = .0475 (from CO_2 analyzer)

Calculate $\dot{V}O_2$, $\dot{V}CO_2$, METs, and R.

Step 1: Calculate $\dot{V}O_2$.

$$\dot{V}O_2 = (\dot{V}I \times FIO_2) - (\dot{V}E \times FEO_2)$$

where

$$\dot{V}I = \frac{\dot{V}E \times FEN_2}{FIN_2 \text{ (constant .7904)}}$$

We now have

$$FEN_2 = 1 - FEO_2 - FECO_2$$
$$FEN_2 = 1 - .1595 - .0475$$
$$FEN_2 = .7930$$
$$\dot{V}I = \frac{72 \text{ L air/min} \times .7930}{.7904}$$
$$\dot{V}I = 72.24 \text{ L air/min}$$

Thus

$$\dot{V}O_2 = (72.24 \text{ L air/min} \times .2093) - (72 \text{ L air/min} \times .1595)$$
$$\dot{V}O_2 = 15.1198 \text{ L } O_2\text{/min} - 11.48 \text{ L } O_2\text{/min}$$
$$\dot{V}O_2 = 3.6 \text{ L } O_2\text{/min or } 3{,}640 \text{ ml } O_2\text{/min}$$

Step 2: Determine MET level.

$$\dot{V}O_2 = \frac{3{,}640 \text{ ml } O_2\text{/min}}{65 \text{ kg}} = 56 \text{ ml } O_2\text{/kg/min}$$

$$\text{METs} = 56 \cancel{\text{ml } O_2\text{/kg/min}} \times \frac{1 \text{ MET}}{3.5 \cancel{\text{ml } O_2\text{/kg/min}}} = 16 \text{ METs}$$

Step 3: Insert the known values into the $\dot{V}CO_2$ equation (equation 2).

$$\dot{V}CO_2 = (\dot{V}E \times FECO_2) - (\dot{V}I \times FICO_2)$$
$$\dot{V}CO_2 = (72 \text{ L air/min} \times .0475) - (72.24 \text{ L air/min} \times .0003)$$
$$\dot{V}CO_2 = 3.42 \text{ L } CO_2\text{/min} - .021672 \text{ L } CO_2\text{/min}$$
$$\dot{V}CO_2 = 3.398328 \text{ L } CO_2\text{/min, rounded off to } 3.40 \text{ L } CO_2\text{/min}$$

Step 4: Determine R.

$$R = \frac{\dot{V}CO_2}{\dot{V}O_2} = \frac{3.40}{3.64} = .934 \text{ rounded to } .93$$

In step 1, using the Haldane equation, we could see that $\dot{V}I$ (72.24 L air/min) was slightly greater than $\dot{V}E$ (72 L air/min). This was a hint that $\dot{V}O_2$ would be slightly greater than $\dot{V}CO_2$, yielding an R value of less than 1.0.

Absolute $\dot{V}O_2$ and Relative $\dot{V}O_2$

In this section you will learn how to convert back and forth between the following:

$$\frac{\text{L } O_2}{\text{min}} \leftrightarrow \frac{\text{ml } O_2}{\text{min}} \leftrightarrow \text{ml } O_2\text{/kg/min}$$

Success with solving all of the workload equations depends upon your ability to quickly make the conversion from liters (L) to milliliters (ml) and to calculate back and forth between an absolute $\dot{V}O_2$ and a relative $\dot{V}O_2$ (i.e., the $\dot{V}O_2$ independent of body weight and the $\dot{V}O_2$ relative to body weight).

Some exercise facilities have open-circuit spirometry equipment for collection and analysis of expired gases. This equipment can analyze expired air and determine an individual's absolute consumption of oxygen (absolute $\dot{V}O_2$) in the units ml O_2/min at rest or during exercise. If you know a subject's body weight you can determine the relative $\dot{V}O_2$, ml O_2/kg/min.

Example 5H

Convert relative $\dot{V}O_2$ to absolute $\dot{V}O_2$. Two subjects, Mary and Tom, are walking on treadmills. They are both walking at 3.65 mph (97.82 m/min) and consuming a relative-to-weight $\dot{V}O_2$ of about 13.28 ml O_2/kg/min. Mary has a body weight of 60 kg, and Tom has a body weight of 90 kg. Determine the absolute $\dot{V}O_2$ and kcal expenditure of both subjects.

Step 1: Determine absolute $\dot{V}O_2$ for each subject. Use a pencil to cancel the unit kg.

(Relative $\dot{V}O_2$) (Absolute $\dot{V}O_2$)

$$\text{Mary: } \frac{13.28 \text{ ml } O_2}{\text{kg/min}} \times 60 \text{ kg} = \frac{796.8 \text{ ml } O_2}{\text{min}}$$

$$\text{Tom: } \frac{13.28 \text{ ml } O_2}{\text{kg/min}} \times 90 \text{ kg} = \frac{1{,}195.2 \text{ ml } O_2}{\text{min}}$$

Tom has a higher absolute $\dot{V}O_2$ at the same walking speed because of his greater number of kilograms of body weight.

Step 2: Calculate each subject's kcal expenditure. Cancel the units so that kcal/min remains as the unit for the answer.

$$\text{Mary: } \frac{796.8 \text{ ml } O_2}{\text{min}} \times \frac{.005 \text{ kcal}}{\text{ml } O_2} = \frac{3.98 \text{ kcal}}{\text{min}}, \text{ almost } \frac{4 \text{ kcal}}{\text{min}}$$

$$\text{Tom: } \frac{1{,}195.2 \text{ ml } O_2}{\text{min}} \times \frac{.005 \text{ kcal}}{\text{ml } O_2} = \frac{5.976 \text{ kcal}}{\text{min}}, \text{ almost } \frac{6 \text{ kcal}}{\text{min}}$$

Tom is consuming 2 kcals/min more than Mary at the same walking speed.

Example 5I will demonstrate the conversion of an absolute $\dot{V}O_2$ to a relative $\dot{V}O_2$.

Example 5I

Convert an absolute $\dot{V}O_2$ to a relative $\dot{V}O_2$. A subject weighs 92 kg and consumes 1,500 ml O_2/min. What is his relative $\dot{V}O_2$?

Step 1: Simply divide the subject's weight in kg into the absolute $\dot{V}O_2$ number. No cancellation is required when you perform this conversion. The unit kg becomes part of the unit ml O_2/kg/min during the process of division.

(Absolute $\dot{V}O_2$) (Relative $\dot{V}O_2$)

$$1{,}500 \text{ ml } O_2/\text{min} \qquad \frac{1{,}500 \text{ ml } O_2/\text{min}}{92 \text{ kg}} = 16 \text{ ml } O_2/\text{kg/min}$$

Summary

The goal of this chapter was to provide the math tools enabling you to gain an understanding of the physiological variables that are measured during a GXT and the numbers and units that you will encounter on exams, during exercise physiology classes at the university level, and at work in the field of exercise science.

Chapter 5 Practice Problems

1. Using Table 5.1, find P H_2O (room) at 23 °C.
2. Using Table 5.1, find P H_2O (lungs) at 37 °C.

In practice questions 3 and 4, round off your *final* answer to two decimal places.

3. Correct the following $\dot{V}E$ from ATPS to BTPS. Use standardization equation B.

   (a) $\dot{V}E \text{ (ATPS)} = \dfrac{7{,}200 \text{ ml air}}{\text{min}}$

   You are given the following information:

   BT = 37 °C
   P H_2O (lungs) = 47 mmHg at the 37 °C body temperature
   AT = 23 °C
   P H_2O (room) = 21 mmHg at 23 °C room temperature
   K = 273 °C
   PB = 752 mmHg wall-mounted barometer

   (b) $\dot{V}E \text{ (ATPS)} = \dfrac{8{,}400 \text{ ml air}}{\text{min}}$

   AT = 21 °C
   All other values are the same as in (a).

   Set up each problem like this: $\dot{V} \times \dfrac{273+}{273+} \times \dfrac{752-}{752-}$

   (c) $\dot{V}E \text{ (ATPS)} = \dfrac{26 \text{ L air}}{\text{min}}$

   Use all of the conditions from (a).

4. Correct a $\dot{V}E$ (BTPS) to $\dot{V}E$ (STPD). Use standardization equation C.

   You are given the following information:

   $\dot{V}E$ (BTPS) = 82 L air/min
   K = 273 °K
   AT = 22 °C
   PB = 750 mmHg
   lung temperature = 37 °C (Use Table 5.1 to determine P H_2O [lungs].)
   SPB = 760 mmHg
   When correcting BTPS to STPD, SPB is used in the equation.
   P H_2O (room) is not found in this equation.

5. Correct a $\dot{V}E$ (BTPS) to $\dot{V}E$ (STPD).

   $\dot{V}E$ (BTPS) = 95 L air/min and AT = 91 °F; use all other values from problem 4.

6. Determine minute ventilation ($\dot{V}E$ in ml air/min) given the following. These values are at BTPS.

	TV	*f*	$\dot{V}E$
(a)	$\dfrac{600 \text{ ml air}}{\text{breath}}$	$\dfrac{12 \text{ breaths}}{\text{min}}$	?
(b)	$\dfrac{750 \text{ ml air}}{\text{breath}}$	$\dfrac{16 \text{ breaths}}{\text{min}}$	?

7. Write out the *unit* for each of the following components, for example, frequency (f) = breaths/min.

   (a) TV = 650

   (b) f = 55

   (c) $\dot{V}E$ = 7,565

8. Determine alveolar ventilation ($\dot{V}A$) using the following information. Which of the following equations is the correct one to use for this problem?

   $\dot{V}A = \dot{V}E - (DS \times f)$

   or

   $\dot{V}A = (TV - DS) \times f$

	$\dot{V}E$ (ml air/min)	DS (ml air/breath)	f (breath/min)
(a)	5,235	165	12
(b)	4,263	142	15
(c)	65,423	175	22

9. Use the following information to solve for physiological dead space. Review Example 5E.

	$\dot{V}E$ (ml air/min)	$\dot{V}A$ (ml air/min)	f (breath/min)
(a)	6,400	3,900	14
(b)	21,400	19,800	12

10. Use the equation $\dot{V}A = (TV - DS) \times f$ to solve for $\dot{V}A$. Physiological DS = anatomical DS.

	TV (ml air/breath)	DS (ml air/breath)	f (breath/min)
(a)	3,000	142	45
(b)	2,000	265	21

11. Choose the correct answer. DS/TV is an indication of

    (a) Ratio of minute ventilation to $\dot{V}A$

    (b) Percent of expiratory volume

    (c) Percent of wasted ventilation

    (d) Ratio of dead space to total ventilation

12. Determine wasted ventilation (DS/TV), ml air/breath.

	Rest	Moderate exercise
(a)	DS = 140 TV = 650	DS = 350 TV = 1,800
(b)	DS = 160 TV = 720	DS = 375 TV = 2,100

13. Identify the $\dot{V}O_2max$ that would most likely represent an elite 10-kilometer distance runner who weighs about 154 lb.

    (a) 80 L O_2/kg/min

    (b) 5 L O_2/min

    (c) 70 to 74 L air/min

    (d) 125 L O_2/min

14. Complete the following Haldane correction equations.

    (a) $\dot{V}I = \dfrac{\dot{V}E \times ?}{?}$

    (b) $\dot{V}E = \dfrac{? \times FIN_2}{?}$

15. When given the following values, determine FEN_2.

	$FECO_2$	FEO_2	FEN_2
(a)	.0455	.1595	?
(b)	.0429	.1599	?
(c)	4.68%	16.52%	?

16. Determine FIN_2 given $FIO_2 = .2093$ and $FECO_2 = .0003$.

    At this point, take a few moments and practice writing down the $\dot{V}O_2$ and $\dot{V}CO_2$ equations. You should be able to write these equations down from memory.

17. A runner has just completed a GXT. Determine the $\dot{V}O_2$ at the end of the test. All values are at STPD conditions. First, list the known values, for example, FIO_2 and $FICO_2$. Second, note that $\dot{V}E$ and $\dot{V}I$ are not equal.

    $FECO_2 = .0450 = 4.5\%$ $\quad$ $\dot{V}I = 100$ L air/min

    $FEO_2 = .1600 = 16.00\%$ $\quad$ $\dot{V}E = 99.42$ L air/min

18. Using the values in question 17, calculate this subject's $\dot{V}CO_2$.

    Use the equation $\dot{V}CO_2 = (\dot{V}E \times FECO_2) - (\dot{V}I \times VICO_2)$.

19. Using $FECO_2 = .0475$, determine $\dot{V}CO_2$ for the following $\dot{V}E$.

    Step 1: List the known values, $FICO_2$ and FIN_2.

    Step 2: Determine FEN_2. $FEO_2 = .1600$

    Use these equations:

    $FEN_2 = 1.00 - FEO_2 - FECO_2$

    and

    $$\dot{V}I = \frac{FEN_2 \times \dot{V}E}{FIN_2}$$

    (a) $\dot{V}E = 95$ L air/min

    (b) $\dot{V}E = 85$ L air/min

(c) $\dot{V}E = 75$ L air/min

20. The following values were recorded during the last minute of a GXT using a cycle ergometer protocol. FIN_2 will always be 79.04%. Determine $\dot{V}O_2$, $\dot{V}CO_2$, and R. First, find $\dot{V}I$ using the Haldane correction equation:

$$\dot{V}I = FEN_2 \times \frac{\dot{V}E}{FIN_2}.$$

$FECO_2 = .0327$

$FEO_2 = .1794$

$\dot{V}E$ (STPD) $= 42$ L air/min

21. A 25-year-old male weighing 70 kg performed a treadmill GXT that was stopped due to exhaustion. Determine the following.

(a) FEN_2

(b) $\dot{V}I$

(c) $\dot{V}O_2$

(d) METs

(e) $\dot{V}CO_2$

(f) Respiratory exchange ratio (R)

The following values were collected during the last minute of the test:

$FECO_2 = .0365$, $FEO_2 = .1785$, and $\dot{V}E$ (STPD) $= 165$ L air/min.

22. The following values were measured during the last minute of GXT performed on a treadmill. Calculate the $\dot{V}O_2$, $\dot{V}CO_2$, and R. $FECO_2 = .0435$; $FEO_2 = .1665$; $\dot{V}E$ (STPD) $= 52$ L air/min.

23. Resting $\dot{V}O_2$ for a healthy 70-kg male is approximately

(a) 62 L air/min

(b) .245 L O_2/min

(c) .5 L air/min

(d) 86 ml O_2/kg/min at a weight of 70 kg

Fill in the blanks where there is a question mark.

24. $\frac{1{,}200 \text{ ml } O_2/\text{min}}{80 \text{ kg}} = ?\ \text{ml } O_2/?/\text{min}$

25. $\frac{1{,}150 \text{ ml } O_2/\text{min}}{65 \text{ kg}} = ?\ ?\ O_2/\text{kg}/\text{min}$

26. $\frac{1{,}420\ ?\ ?/\text{min}}{70\ ?} = ?\ \text{ml } O_2/\text{kg}/?$

Convert $\frac{\text{L } O_2}{\text{min}} \leftrightarrow \frac{\text{ml } O_2}{\text{min}}$ in problems 27 through 33.

27. $3 \text{ L } O_2 \text{ min}^{-1} = \frac{?\ \text{L } O_2}{\text{min}}$

$$\frac{3\ L\ O_2}{min} \times \frac{1{,}000\ ml}{1\ L} = ?\ \frac{ml\ O_2}{min}$$

28. $\frac{5\ L\ O_2}{min} \times \frac{1{,}000\ ml}{1\ L} = ?$ (Include the units in the answer.)

29. $\frac{2.5\ L\ O_2}{min} \times \frac{1{,}000\ ml}{1\ L} = ?$

30. $\frac{5{,}500\ ml\ O_2}{min} \times \frac{1\ L}{1{,}000\ ml} = \frac{?\ L\ O_2}{min}$

31. $\frac{4{,}800\ ml\ O_2}{min} \times ? = \frac{?\ L\ O_2}{min}$

32. $4.5\ L\ O_2\ min^{-1} = ?$

33. $\frac{3.6\ L\ O_2}{min} = \frac{?\ ml\ O_2}{min}$

Perform the following. Write out all of the units as you perform these problems.

34. With a subject's weight at 70 kg, convert 4.5 L O_2/min to ml O_2/min, and then to a relative $\dot{V}O_2$ (ml O_2/kg/min).
35. Subject's weight = 80 kg. Convert 4.0 L O_2/min to ml O_2/min and then to the units ml O_2/kg/min.
36. Convert the following relative-to-weight $\dot{V}O_2$ values to absolute $\dot{V}O_2$ values. Subject's weight is 70 kg.
    (a) $\frac{49\ ml\ O_2}{kg/min}$
    (b) 42 ml O_2/kg/min
    (c) 36 ml O_2/kg/min

Chapter 5 Answers to Practice Problems

1. 21 mmHg
2. 47 mmHg
3. ATPS corrected to BTPS

   (a) $\dot{V}E\ (ATPS) = \frac{7{,}200\ ml\ air}{min}$: correcting to $\dot{V}E$ (BTPS)

$$\frac{7{,}200\ ml\ air}{min} \times \frac{K + BT}{K + AT} \times \frac{P_B - P\ H_2O\ (room)}{P_B - P\ H_2O\ (lungs)} = \dot{V}E\ (BTPS)$$

$$\frac{7{,}200\ ml\ air}{min} \times \frac{273\ °K + 37\ °C}{273\ °K + 23\ °C} \times \frac{752\ mmHg - 21\ mmHg}{752\ mmHg - 47\ mmHg} = \dot{V}E\ (BTPS)$$

$$\frac{7{,}200\ ml\ air}{min} \times \frac{310\ °K}{296\ °K} \times \frac{731\ \cancel{mmHg}}{705\ \cancel{mmHg}} = \dot{V}E\ (BTPS)$$

$$\frac{7{,}200\ ml\ air}{min} \times 1.0472972 \times 1.0368794 = \dot{V}E\ (BTPS)$$

$$7{,}818.6297 = \frac{7{,}818.63\ ml\ air}{min} = \dot{V}E\ (BTPS)$$

Remember, when correcting from ATPS to BTPS, a volume increases.

(b) $\dot{V}E\ (ATPS) = \dfrac{8{,}400 \text{ ml air}}{\text{min}}$ corrected to $\dot{V}E\ (BTPS) = \dfrac{9{,}183.79 \text{ ml air}}{\text{min}}$

Math check: $8{,}400 \times 1.0544217 \times 1.0368794 = 9{,}183.7882$

(c) $\dot{V}E\ (ATPS) = \dfrac{26 \text{ L air}}{\text{min}}$ corrected to $\dot{V}E\ (BTPS) = \dfrac{28.23 \text{ L air}}{\text{min}}$

Math check: $26 \times 1.0472972 \times 1.0368794 = 28.23394$

4. $\dot{V}E$ (BTPS) = 82 L air/min is corrected to

   $\dot{V}E$ (STPD) = 70.19 L air/min. The volume decreases.

   Math check: $82 \times .9254237 \times .925 = 70.193387$

5. $\dot{V}E$ (BTPS) of 95 L air/min is corrected to

   $\dot{V}E$ (STPD) = 78.4 L air/min. The volume decreases.

   Math check: $95 \times .8921568 \times .925 = 78.398278$

6. (a) $\dot{V}E = TV \times f$

   $$\dot{V}E = \frac{600 \text{ ml air}}{\cancel{\text{breath}}} \times \frac{12\ \cancel{\text{breaths}}}{\text{min}}$$

   $$\dot{V}E = \frac{7{,}200 \text{ ml air}}{\text{min}}$$

   (b) $\dot{V}E$ = 12,000 ml air/min

7. Units

   (a) $TV = \dfrac{650 \text{ ml air}}{\text{breath}}$

   (b) f = 55 breaths/min

   (c) $\dot{V}E$ = 7,565 ml air/min

8. $\dot{V}A = \dot{V}E - (DS \times f)$

   (a) $\dot{V}A$ = 3,255 ml air/min

   (b) $\dot{V}A$ = 2,133 ml air/min

   (c) $\dot{V}A$ = 61,573 ml air/min

9. Physiological DS (Note: $\dot{V}A$ will always be smaller than $\dot{V}E$.)

   (a) 178.57 ml air/breath

   (b) 133.33 ml air/breath

10. $\dot{V}A$ (ml of air that ventilates alveoli)

   (a) 128,610 ml air/min or 128 L air/min

   (b) 36,435 ml air/min

11. DS/TV = (c) percent of wasted ventilation.
12. DS/TV

	Rest	Moderate exercise
(a)	21.54%	19.44%
(b)	22.22%	17.86%

Note: In healthy subjects DS/TV ratio decreases with exercise.

13. (b) 5 L O_2/min
14. (a) $\dot{V}I = \dfrac{\dot{V}E \times FEN_2}{FIN_2}$

    (b) $\dot{V}E = \dfrac{\dot{V}I \times FIN_2}{FEN_2}$
15. FEN_2
    (a) .7950
    (b) .7972
    (c) .7880
16. FIN_2 = 79.04%; FIN_2 will always be .7904.
17. $\dot{V}O_2 = (\dot{V}I \times FIO_2) - (\dot{V}E \times FEO_2)$
    $\dot{V}O_2$ = (100 L air/min × .2093) − (99.42 L air/min × .1600)
    $\dot{V}O_2$ = 20.93 L O_2/min − 15.9072 L O_2/min
    $\dot{V}O_2$ = 5.02 L O_2/min

    Hint: Review Example 5G.
18. $\dot{V}CO_2$ = 4.4739 − .03 = 4.44 L CO_2/min
19. $\dot{V}CO_2$ in L/min   Math check:
    (a) 4.48 = (95 × .0475) − (95.252403 × .0003)
    (b) 4.01 = (85 × .0475) − (85.225835 × .0003)
    (c) 3.54 = (75 × .0475) − (75.199266 × .0003)
20. FEN_2 = .7879 $\dot{V}I$ = 41.867155 L air/min
    $\dot{V}O_2$ = 1.23 L O_2/min = (41.867155 × .2093) − (42 × .1794)
    $\dot{V}CO_2$ = 1.36 L CO_2/min = (42 × .0327) − (41.867155 × .0003)
21. (a) FEN_2 = .7850
    (b) $\dot{V}I$ = 163.87272 L air/min
    (c) $\dot{V}O_2$ = 34.3 − 29.45 = 4.85 L O_2/min
    (d) METs = 19.8
    (e) $\dot{V}CO_2$ = 5.973 L CO_2/min
    (f) R = 1.23
22. FEN_2 = .7900 $\dot{V}I$ = 51.973684

$\dot{V}O_2 = 2.22 \text{ L } O_2/\text{min}$

$\dot{V}CO_2 = 2.25 \text{ L } CO_2/\text{min}$

$R = 1.01$

23. (b) .245 L O_2/min

24. $\dfrac{1{,}200 \text{ ml } O_2/\text{min}}{80 \text{ kg}} = 15 \text{ ml } O_2/\text{kg}/\text{min}$

25. $\dfrac{1{,}150 \text{ ml } O_2/\text{min}}{65 \text{ kg}} = 17.69 \text{ ml } O_2/\text{kg}/\text{min}$

26. $\dfrac{1{,}420 \text{ ml } O_2/\text{min}}{70 \text{ kg}} = 20.29 \text{ ml } O_2/\text{kg}/\text{min}$

27. $3 \text{ L } O_2 \text{ min}^{-1} = \dfrac{3 \text{ L } O_2}{\text{min}}$

$$\frac{3 \not{\text{L}}\ O_2}{\text{min}} \times \frac{1{,}000 \text{ ml}}{1 \not{\text{L}}} = \frac{3{,}000 \text{ ml } O_2}{\text{min}}$$

28. $\dfrac{5 \not{\text{L}}\ O_2}{\text{min}} \times \dfrac{1{,}000}{1 \not{\text{L}}} = 5{,}000 \text{ ml } O_2/\text{min}$

29. $\dfrac{2.5 \not{\text{L}}\ O_2}{\text{min}} \times \dfrac{1{,}000 \text{ ml}}{1 \not{\text{L}}} = 2{,}500 \text{ ml } O_2/\text{min}$

30. $\dfrac{5{,}500 \not{\text{ml}}\, O_2}{\text{min}} \times \dfrac{1 \text{ L}}{1{,}000 \not{\text{ml}}} = \dfrac{5.50 \text{ L } O_2}{\text{min}}$

31. $\dfrac{4{,}800 \not{\text{ml}}\, O_2}{\text{min}} \times \dfrac{1 \text{ L}}{1{,}000 \not{\text{ml}}} = \dfrac{4.80 \text{ L } O_2}{\text{min}}$

32. $4.50 \text{ L } O_2 \text{ min}^{-1} = 4.50 \text{ L } O_2/\text{min}$

33. $\dfrac{3.60 \text{ L } O_2}{\text{min}} = \dfrac{3{,}600 \text{ ml } O_2}{\text{min}}$

34. $4.5 \text{ L } O_2/\text{min} = 4{,}500 \text{ ml } O_2/\text{min}$

$$\frac{4{,}500 \text{ ml } O_2/\text{min}}{70 \text{ kg}} = 64.29 \text{ ml } O_2/\text{kg}/\text{min}$$

35. $4.0 \text{ L } O_2/\text{min} = 4{,}000 \text{ ml } O_2/\text{min} = 50 \text{ ml } O_2/\text{kg}/\text{min}$

36. (a) $\dfrac{49 \text{ ml } O_2}{\text{kg}/\text{min}} \times 70 \text{ kg} = 3{,}430 \text{ ml } O_2/\text{min}$ = an absolute $\dot{V}O_2$

(b) 2,940 ml O_2/min

(c) 2,520 ml O_2/min

6 Resting Energy Expenditure and Bayes Theorem

Major Concepts

Resting energy expenditure

Converting METs to kcal

Bayes theorem, specificity, sensitivity

Karvonen formula and training heart rate (THR)

Resting Oxygen Uptake and Resting Energy Expenditure

Resting oxygen uptake is defined as the amount of oxygen consumed while at rest, also referred to as resting metabolic rate (RMR) or resting energy expenditure (REE) (Howley & Franks, 1992; Zavala, 1987, 1989). There are several ways, such as direct calorimetry, to measure RMR. RMR can also be measured directly via oxygen consumption. There is a direct relationship between oxygen consumption and caloric expenditure; for every liter of oxygen consumed, approximately 5 kcal of energy are expended.

REE is approximately 10% greater than basal metabolic rate (BMR). Measurement of BMR requires that the following conditions be met:

- The subject must spend the night in the laboratory, and is measured immediately upon wakening.
- The subject must fast for 12 hr prior to the measurement.
- All physical and psychological factors of excitement must be removed.
- Room temperature must be 68–80 °F (ACSM, 1988; Guyton, 1991).

Measurement of RMR, on the other hand, can be performed 3 to 4 hr following a meal and after just 30 min of quiet resting in a supine position. For practical reasons RMR rather than BMR is usually measured.

Since it is not always feasible to measure REE or RMR directly, an estimation can be performed using the Harris-Benedict equation. This commonly used equation estimates a subject's resting energy expenditure for a 24-hr period. Body weight, age, and height are used to compute this value (Zavala, 1989). The equation for males is

$$\frac{\text{kcal}}{24\text{ hr}} = [66.473 + (13.752 \times \text{wt}) + (5.003 \times \text{ht})] - (6.755 \times \text{age})$$

The equation for females is

$$\frac{\text{kcal}}{24\text{ hr}} = [655.096 + (9.563 \times \text{wt}) + (1.85 \times \text{ht})] - (4.676 \times \text{age})$$

As you can see in the equations, the REE depends a great deal upon body weight; this factor is more important than age or height. It should also be noted that energy expenditures at rest decrease with age.

As you work through Examples 6A and 6B you will notice how the constants in each equation influence the REE. You will notice that the unit kcal is used rather than cal, or calories.

Example 6A

Determine REE for a female. A 40-year-old female is 172 cm tall and weighs 68 kg. Find her REE.

Step 1: Put known values into the equation.

$$\frac{\text{kcal}}{24\text{ hr}} = [655.096 + (9.563 \times 68\text{ kg}) + (1.85 \times 172\text{ cm})] - (4.676 \times 40\text{ years})$$

Step 2: Perform the math.

$$\frac{\text{kcal}}{24\text{ hr}} = [655.096 + 650.284 + 318.2] - (187.04)$$

$$\frac{\text{kcal}}{24\text{ hr}} = 1{,}623.58 - (187.04)$$

$$\frac{\text{kcal}}{24\text{ hr}} = 1{,}436.54\text{ kcal/24 hr, rounded to }1{,}437\text{ kcal/24 hr,}$$

or approximately 60 kcal/hr

Example 6B

Determine REE for a male. A 40-year-old man is 68 in tall and weighs 150 lb. Find his REE.

Step 1: Convert lb to kg and in to cm.

$$150\text{ lb} \times \frac{1\text{ kg}}{2.2\text{ lb}} = 68\text{ kg}$$

$$68\text{ inch} \times \frac{2.54\text{ cm}}{1\text{ in}} = 172\text{ cm}$$

Step 2: Put known values into the equation.

$$\frac{\text{kcal}}{24\text{ hr}} = [66.473 + (13.752 \times 68\text{ kg}) + (5.003 \times 172\text{ cm})] - (6.755 \times 40\text{ years})$$

Step 3: Perform the math.

$$\frac{\text{kcal}}{24\text{ hr}} = [66.473 + 935.136 + 860.516] - (270.20)$$

$$\frac{\text{kcal}}{24\text{ hr}} = 1{,}862.125 - 270.20$$

$$\frac{\text{kcal}}{24\text{ hr}} = 1{,}591.925\text{ kcal/24 hr, rounded to 1,592 kcal/hr,}$$

or approximately 66 kcal per hour.

You will notice that we compared a man and a woman of the same weight, height, and age. The REE is about 10% higher for males than for females due to a higher percent body fat in females. When metabolic rate is expressed per unit of lean tissue there is little or no difference between men and women (McArdle et al., 1994; Wilmore, 1982).

Converting METs to kcal

The math of converting METs (metabolic equivalents) to kcal is being presented as a separate section in this text because of its importance. Determination of a subject's MET level (ACSM, 1995) is often the final math calculation in metabolic problems dealing with energy expenditure ($\dot{V}O_2$), as you will see in chapters 7 through 12.

The next logical step after determining METs is to specify the kcal expenditure at this level of effort.

Many people use exercise as a means of reducing their percentage of body fat. When exercise intensity is known and there is no change in kilocalorie intake, we can closely estimate how many minutes, weeks, or months would be required to metabolize a given amount of body fat. Examples 6C, 6D, and 6E will illustrate methods for determining kcal expenditure based upon METs and the length and number of workout sessions.

Example 6C

Convert METs into kcals expended. Kristi, who weighs 70 kg, exercises for 48 min at 9 METs each workout. How many kcals does she expend in that 48-min period? Use your calculator to follow the steps through this example. Use the conversion factors

$$\frac{1\text{ kcal/kg/hr}}{1\text{ MET}} \text{ and } \frac{1\text{ hr}}{60\text{ min}}$$

Step 1: Convert METs into kcal/kg/hr.

$$9\,\cancel{\text{METs}} \times \frac{1\text{ kcal/kg/hr}}{1\,\cancel{\text{MET}}} = 9\text{ kcal/kg/hr} = \frac{9\text{ kcal}}{\text{kg/hr}}$$

Step 2: Convert the kcal/kg/hr to kcal/hr.

$$\frac{9\text{ kcal}}{\cancel{\text{kg}}/\text{hr}} \times 70\ \cancel{\text{kg}} = \frac{630\text{ kcal}}{1\text{ hr}}$$

Step 3: Convert kcal/hr to kcal/min.

$$\frac{630\text{ kcal}}{1\ \cancel{\text{hr}}} \times \frac{1\ \cancel{\text{hr}}}{60\text{ min}} = \frac{10.5\text{ kcal}}{\text{min}}$$

Step 4: Convert kcal/min to kcal/workout. In this case, 48 min/workout is the conversion factor.

$$\frac{10.5\text{ kcal}}{\cancel{\text{min}}} \times \frac{48\ \cancel{\text{min}}}{\text{workout}} = \frac{504\text{ kcal}}{\text{workout}}$$

A 70-kg subject expends 504 kcal during a 48-min, 9-MET workout.

Example 6D

Determine how many workouts are needed to expend a given number of kcal. From Example 6C, our female exerciser is using 504 kcal/workout. With three workouts per week, how many weeks will it take to expend 7,000 kcal?

Step 1: Convert kcal/workout to kcal/week.

$$\frac{504\text{ kcal}}{\cancel{\text{workout}}} \times \frac{3\ \cancel{\text{workouts}}}{\text{week}} = \frac{1{,}512\text{ kcal}}{1\text{ week}}$$

Step 2: Convert the 7,000 kcal to weeks.

$$7{,}000\ \cancel{\text{kcal}} \times \frac{1\text{ week}}{1{,}512\ \cancel{\text{kcal}}} = 4.63\text{ weeks, almost 5 weeks, or about 15 workouts}$$

A 70-kg female exercising at 9 METs for 48 min three times per week will be able to expend 7,000 kcal in 15 exercise sessions, or in about 5 weeks; 7,000 kcal represents about 2 lb of fat.

In Example 6C we used the conversion factor 1 MET = 1 kcal/kg/hr. In Example 6E we will use 1 MET = 3.5 ml O_2/kg/min and .005 kcal = 1 ml O_2 as the conversion factors. When familiar with the units and calculations in this section you will be able to solve a wide variety of math problems that involve METs and kcals.

Example 6E

Determine number of kcals expended in a given time at a given intensity. Meredith, who weighs 59 kg, exercised for 8 min at an intensity of 6 METs. How many kcal did she expend?

Step 1: Convert METs to ml O_2/kg/min.

$$6\ \cancel{\text{METs}} \times \frac{3.5\text{ ml }O_2\text{ kg/min}}{1\ \cancel{\text{MET}}} = 21\text{ ml }O_2\text{/kg/min} = \frac{21\text{ ml }O_2}{\text{kg/min}}$$

Step 2: Use the subject's weight to convert the relative VO_2 to an absolute $\dot{V}O_2$.

$$\underset{\text{(Relative)}}{\frac{21 \text{ ml } O_2}{\cancel{\text{kg}}/\text{min}}} \times 59 \cancel{\text{kg}} = \underset{\text{(Absolute)}}{\frac{1{,}239 \text{ ml } O_2}{\text{min}}}$$

Step 3: Convert the relative $\dot{V}O_2$ to kcal/min.
Use .005 kcal = 1 ml O_2 as the conversion factor. The unit ml O_2 cancels.

$$\frac{1{,}239 \cancel{\text{ml } O_2}}{\text{min}} \times \frac{.005 \text{ kcal}}{1 \cancel{\text{ml } O_2}} = \frac{6.195 \text{ kcal}}{\text{min}}$$

Step 4: Determine the total kcal expended in 8 min.

$$\frac{6.195 \text{ kcal}}{\cancel{\text{min}}} \times 8 \cancel{\text{min}} = 49.56 \text{ kcal, approximately 50 kcal in 8 min}$$

Bayesian Analysis (Bayes Theorem)

Bayes theorem is a mathematical calculation used to determine the posttest probability of disease when certain information is known:

- The pretest likelihood of disease
- The sensitivity of a diagnostic test
- The specificity of a diagnostic test.

In short, Bayes theorem implies that the probability of disease after a GXT depends on the pretest probability of disease and the specificity and sensitivity of the GXT based on ST segment depression of 1 mm or greater.

The discussion here will provide the basic concepts and mathematics of Bayes theorem. You can find more information on Bayes theorem in other sources if you are interested (ACSM, 1988; Ellestad, 1986; Epstein, 1979, 1980; Froelicher, 1973, 1987, and 1989; Goldberger, 1991; Griner, 1980; Jones, 1988; Sox, 1988; Weiner et al., 1979; Weinstein, 1980).

Applied to medicine, Bayes theorem is used to identify circumstances in which physicians can use results of selected diagnostic tests to appropriately treat patients. Although the discussion here centers on the graded exercise test electrocardiogram, Bayes' theorem can be used with many other diagnostic tests, including enzyme assays for diagnosis of heart attack, X rays, and glucose tolerance tests (Sox, 1988).

To understand how Bayes theorem is used in interpreting the results of various diagnostic tests, you need to understand the concepts of true and false positivity and negativity. If during a GXT someone exercises to the point of exhaustion with normal ECG and blood pressure responses and no symptoms, the GXT is considered *negative.* If, however, even one of the listed values is abnormal, then the evaluation is a *positive GXT.* For example, a positive GXT would result if the attending physician terminated the test due to such indicators as 2 mm or greater ST segment depression, a series of premature ventricular contractions (PVCs), or a report from the patient of chest and jaw anginal discomfort. To be judged positive, an ST segment depression must reach 1 mm or greater (Epstein, 1980; Weiner et al., 1979). Many physicians will not terminate a GXT until the ST segment reaches 2 to 4 mm of depression; ACSM (1995) suggests termination at 4 mm or greater ST segment depression. A GXT may also be labeled positive if abnormalities occur at $\dot{V}O_2max$ or during initial recovery.

In the case of a false positive GXT, the GXT is positive, but on further evaluation with an invasive procedure (thallium scan) the patient is found not to have disease. Several factors may be reasons for false positive GXT results. With a false negative GXT, the GXT is negative but the patient is found on further evaluation to have disease. A GXT can be false negative for a host of reasons, including stopping the test too soon, failure to identify disease indicators, and technical error.

Evaluation of ST Segment To Be Used in the Bayes Theorem

The reason for performing a GXT is the evaluation of ST segment ECG changes during increasing workloads, which is an indicator of coronary artery disease (CAD). The physician is interested in the diagnostic value of a GXT. The GXT represents a noninvasive, less costly alternative to the use of thallium studies or echocardiograms. However, the ability of the GXT to accurately identify CAD is less than perfect. The question being asked is, what is the probability of a patient's having a diagnosis of CAD based on the results of the GXT coupled with the pretest likelihood of CAD? Bayes theorem can assist in answering this question.

Accuracy of the Graded Exercise Test

Because the accuracy of the GXT is less than 100%, additional information is needed to increase the probability that the GXT results truly identify CAD. For this reason pretest information based upon a patient's symptoms, age, and gender are considered along with the results of the GXT electrocardiogram (ECG).

The accuracy of a GXT with CAD patients is defined by the test's specificity and sensitivity. The results from coronary angiography (X ray view of the coronary arteries) are used as the gold standard for comparison with the GXT. There are four possible outcomes for the GXT:

- True positive—The test is positive and the patient has CAD.
- True negative—The test is negative and the patient does not have CAD.
- False positive—The test is positive but the patient does not have CAD.
- False negative—The test is negative but the patient has CAD.

Specificity and Sensitivity

Knowing the outcome of the GXT and the disease status of the group in which the test was conducted allows calculation of the test sensitivity and specificity.

Specificity Specificity indicates the ability of a GXT to identify healthy subjects when all subjects are truly healthy, that is, the percentage of normal subjects who have negative tests. The following equation is used to determine percentage of specificity of a GXT.

$$\text{Specificity} = \frac{\text{\# of true negative tests}}{\text{\# of true negative tests} + \text{\# of false positive tests}} \times 100\%$$

Example 6F illustrates solving for specificity of a GXT.

Example 6F

Determine GXT specificity. The Bruce protocol treadmill GXT was used to test 20 healthy subjects. Eighteen tests were true negative and two tests were false positive. Determine specificity.

Step 1: Put the known values into the equation and do the math.

$$\text{Specificity} = \frac{18}{18 + 2} \times 100\% = 90\% = .90$$

This GXT, with the given population did its job 90% of the time. Two subjects of the 20 were falsely identified as having CAD when in fact they were healthy.

Sensitivity The sensitivity of a GXT indicates its accuracy for detecting CAD in a group of subjects who all have CAD:

$$\text{Sensitivity} = \frac{\text{\# of true positive tests}}{\text{\# of true positive tests} + \text{\# of false negative tests}} \times 100\%$$

This equation is used to calculate the sensitivity of a GXT used with a certain population of subjects. Example 6G provides an illustration.

Example 6G

Determine GXT sensitivity. The Balke protocol treadmill test was performed on 20 subjects who all had documented CAD. Nineteen were true positive tests (truly abnormal) and one was false negative. Determine sensitivity.

Step 1: Put the known values into the equation and perform the math.

$$\text{Sensitivity} = \frac{19}{19 + 1} \times 100\% = 95\% = .95$$

In this example the GXT did its job at identifying CAD 95% of the time. Most studies that have been completed to determine specificity and sensitivity for a GXT have used very large populations of several hundred subjects (Froelicher, 1973; Rifkin & Hood, 1977; Weiner et al., 1979). In examples 6F and 6G, small population numbers (20) were used to demonstrate the concepts of specificity and sensitivity.

The specificity and sensitivity of a GXT differ depending on the pretest probability of CAD in the population under study. When studying the examples and performing the practice problems in this section be aware of the slightly different specificity and sensitivity values.

Several authors (Diamond & Forrester, 1979; Epstein, 1980; Rifkin & Hood, 1977; Weiner et al., 1979) have presented complex mathematical equations, based upon age, gender, and symptoms, to calculate pretest (pre-GXT) likelihood of CAD. Fortunately for us, Diamond and Forrester (1979) have already calculated a wide variety of combinations of age, gender, and symptoms to compile a table of pretest likelihood percentages (pp. 1352, 1354). Table 6.1 is an adaptation from the figures presented by Diamond and Forrester (1979), and can also be found in ACSM (1988, p. 226). Rather than calculating pretest likelihood of CAD we will refer here to Table 6.1 for the likelihood percentages. Examination of Table 6.1 reveals three trends of CAD:

- Likelihood percentage increases with age.
- Likelihood percentage increases with the severity of anginal symptoms.
- Men have a higher likelihood percentage than women.

Use table 6.1 to solve the problems that follow.

Table 6.1 Pretest Likelihood Percentages (%) of Coronary Artery Disease in Symptomatic and Asymptomatic Subjects According to Age and Gender

Age (average)	Asymptomatic		Non-anginal chest pain		Atypical angina[a]		Typical angina[b]	
	Men	Women	Men	Women	Men	Women	Men	Women
30–39 (35)	1.9	0.3	5.2	0.8	21.8	4.2	69.7	25.8
40–49 (45)	5.5	1.0	14.1	2.8	46.1	13.3	87.3	55.2
50–59 (55)	9.7	3.2	21.5	8.4	58.9	32.4	92.0	79.4
60–69 (65)	12.3	7.5	28.1	18.6	67.1	54.4	94.3	90.6

[a]Atypical angina: chest pain that is not associated with the classic symptoms of typical angina. This pain may be sharp and short in duration, for example, may or may not occur with exercise, and does not including sweating, nausea, etc.
[b]Typical angina: pressure-type pain in the chest, shoulders, neck, or jaw area, perhaps radiating to the arms, that occurs with exercise or emotional stress. This type of angina may be associated with sweating, nausea, and weakness and is relieved by taking nitroglycerin medication.
From "Additional Diagnostic Tests: Special Populations," by B. A. Franklin, V. Hollingsworth, and L. M. Borysyk. In *Resource Manual for Guidelines for Exercise Testing and Prescription* (p. 226) by American College of Sports Medicine, 1988, Philadelphia: Lea & Febiger. Copyright 1988 by Lea & Febiger. Reprinted with permission.
Franklin, et al table adapted from "Analysis of Probability as an Aid in the Clinical Diagnosis of Coronary-Artery Disease" by G. A. Diamond and J. S. Forrester, 1979, *New England Journal of Medicine*, **300**, p. 1350. Copyright 1979. Adapted with permission.

Problem 1: What is the pretest likelihood percentage of a subject who is male, 45 years old, and experiencing atypical angina?

Answer: 46.1% pretest likelihood of CAD

Problem 2: Identify the pretest likelihood percentage of a female subject, age 65, who experiences typical anginal symptoms.

Answer: 90.6% pretest likelihood of CAD

Problem 3: List three subjects who have a 12% to 15% pretest likelihood of coronary artery disease.

Answer:
1. Male, age 65, asymptomatic
2. Male, age 45, non-anginal chest pain
3. Female, age 45, atypical angina

Putting Bayes Theorem All Together

The posttest probability of CAD can be calculated from the pretest likelihood of CAD, the test specificity and sensitivity, and the outcome of the GXT (positive or negative). If the GXT is negative the posttest probability of CAD can calculated:

Posttest probability (negative test)

$$= \frac{\text{pretest probability} \times (1 - \text{sensitivity})}{\text{pretest probability} \times (1 - \text{sensitivity}) + (1 - \text{pretest probability})(\text{specificity})}$$

If the GXT is positive, the posttest probability is

Posttest probability (positive test)

$$= \frac{\text{pretest probability of CAD (\%)} \times \text{sensitivity}}{\text{pretest probability} \times \text{sensitivity} + (1 - \text{pretest probability})(1 - \text{specificity})}$$

The next three examples use Bayes theorem to calculate the posttest probability of CAD. Please note the differences in sensitivity and specificity for GXTs when used in different populations.

Example 6H

Determine posttest probability for CAD. A 65-year-old male is experiencing atypical angina. His GXT revealed positive results with 2 mm ST segment depression. Test sensitivity is 70% and specificity is 90%. Calculate posttest probability for CAD.

Step 1: Find the pretest likelihood percentage from Table 6.1.
Pretest likelihood = 67.1% (rounded off to 67%).

Step 2: Determine which posttest probability equation to use.
Because GXT was positive, we use the positive equation.

Step 3: Enter the known values into the equation and perform the math.

$$\text{Posttest probability (pos)} = \frac{.67 \times .70}{(.67 \times .70) + (1 - .67)(1 - .90)}$$

$$\text{Posttest probability (pos)} = \frac{.469}{.469 + .033}$$

$$\text{Posttest probability (pos)} = \frac{.469}{.502} = 93\% \text{ probability of CAD}$$

A posttest probability of 93% for CAD after a positive GXT is consistent with a pretest likelihood of 67%.

Example 6I

Determine posttest probability of CAD. A 65-year-old female is experiencing non-anginal chest pain. Her Balke protocol treadmill GXT was negative for ST segment changes. GXT sensitivity is 70% and specificity is 90%. Calculate the posttest probability of CAD.

Step 1: Find the pretest sensitivity from Table 6.1.
Pretest sensitivity is 18.6%.

Step 2: Determine which posttest probability equation to use.
The GXT was negative, so we must use the negative test equation.

Step 3: Enter the known values into the equation and perform the math.

$$\text{Posttest probability (neg)} = \frac{.186 \times (1 - .70)}{.186 \times (1 - .70) + (1 - .186)(.90)}$$

$$\text{Posttest probability (neg)} = \frac{.0558}{.7884} = .07 = 7\% \text{ probability of CAD}$$

When the pretest likelihood of CAD is known, a graph can be created by plotting points based on specificity and sensitivity. The graph can then be used instead of the equations to determine the posttest probability of CAD. Figure 6.1 is an example of a graph based on a GXT with a sensitivity of 75% and specificity of 85% (Epstein, 1980). To use the graph, find the pretest likelihood of CAD on the bottom axis. Draw a line straight up from that percentage. If the subject has a negative GXT, note where the line you drew crosses the negative GXT curve. Draw a line from the intersection to the vertical axis. The point at which the line crosses the vertical axis indicates the percentage of posttest probability of CAD. If the subject has a positive GXT, repeat the process using the intersection of the line from the horizontal axis and the positive GXT curve.

Example 6J

Determine posttest probability of CAD from a graph. A 65-year-old female subject has a pretest likelihood of 54.4% of CAD. Using Figure 6.1, determine posttest likelihood of CAD if her GXT was negative, and then if her GXT was positive.

Step 1: Find the pretest likelihood of CAD on the horizontal axis of the graph in Figure 6.1.
Pretest likelihood is 54.4%.

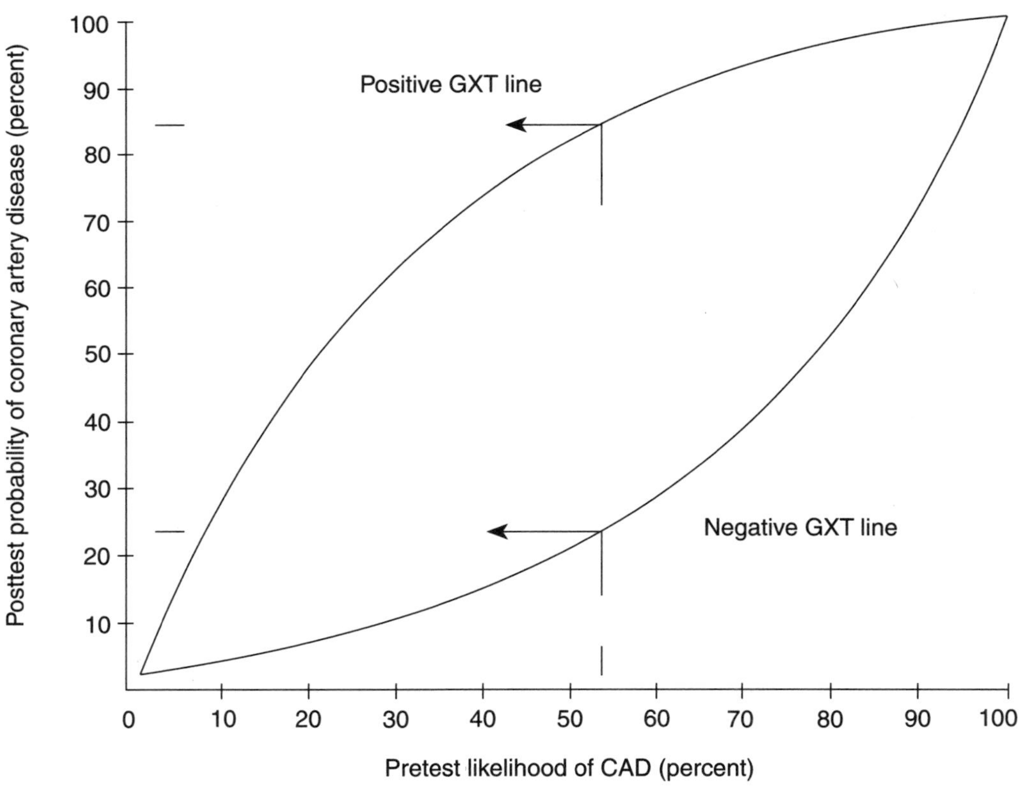

Figure 6.1 Determination of posttest probability of CAD when pretest likelihood is known (based on a GXT with a sensitivity of 75% and specificity of 85%).
From "Implications of Probability Analysis on the Strategy Used for Noninvasive Detection of Coronary Artery Disease," by S. E. Epstein, 1980, *The American Journal of Cardiology*, **46 (3)**, p. 493. Copyright 1980. Reprinted with permission.

Step 2: Draw a line up from 54.4% to the point of intersection with the negative GXT line. Continue the line to the point of intersection with the positive GXT line.

Step 3: Draw lines from the points of intersection to the vertical axis.

Step 4: Note the percentage values indicated by the intersection of the lines you drew and the vertical axis. These are the posttest probabilities of CAD.
Posttest probability of CAD for subject with negative GXT = 24%
Posttest probability of CAD for subject with positive GXT = 85%

Determining Appropriate Exercise Intensity

An exercise prescription requires a mode (cycle, arm ergometer, treadmill, walking, etc.), a duration (number of minutes), a frequency (number of days per week), and a prescribed intensity.

Ascertaining the correct intensity is important because the subject must exercise with enough effort to receive at least minimal cardiovascular conditioning effects, while at the same time minimizing the possibility of musculoskeletal injury, cardiorespiratory complications, excess fatigue, or a prolonged recovery period.

The lower limit of prescribed exercise intensity is as important as the upper intensity. Exercising at an intensity consistent with 60% to 80% of $\dot{V}O_2max$ and the corresponding heart rate (HR) has been shown to provide the best range for developing cardiovascular benefits for the normal healthy adult (ACSM, 1988; Bouchard, Shephard, Stephens, Sutton, & McPherson, 1990).

In some cases, exercising below 60% of measured or predicted $\dot{V}O_2max$ or HRmax (220 − age) is appropriate. A sedentary person whose daily effort level is no more than 30% of the predicted HRmax will receive cardiovascular benefits at an intensity of 40% of HRmax. When cardiovascular conditioning has improved over a period of training, the prescribed training HR range can be recalculated.

Using $\dot{V}O_2$

The most direct method to establish exercise intensity is to use the HR and O_2 consumption values from a GXT. Heart rate and O_2 consumption increase linearly with increasing work. The HR that corresponds to the recommended exercise intensity for apparently healthy adults (60–80% VO_2max) can be measured and used to monitor exercise sessions. However, measuring HR and VO_2 during a GXT is impractical in many situations. Therefore, alternative methods to establish training heart rate ranges have been developed.

The Karvonen Formula

The Karvonen formula can be used to determine training heart rate (THR) based upon a percentage of the heart rate reserve (HRR). The HRR is the difference between the maximal HR and the HR at rest. Maximal HR can be measured during an exercise test or estimated from the formula HRmax = 220 − age. Resting HR can be measured for 1 min upon awakening in the morning or following 15 min of sitting or lying quietly.

The upper and lower bounds of the THR range are calculated as follows:

THR (lower bound) = (HRmax − HRrest) × .60 (or derived lowest intensity) + HRrest

THR (upper bound) = (HRmax − HRrest) × .85 (or derived highest intensity) + HRrest

The following examples illustrate the use of the Karvonen formula.

Example 6K

Calculate THR with the Karvonen formula. Mr. Jones (age 30 years) achieved a maximum heart rate of 195 beats/min during a GXT. His heart rate at rest was 55 bt/min. Mr. Jones should exercise at 60% to 80% of HRmax. Calculate his THR.

Step 1: Calculate the lower bound.

THR (lower bound) = (HRmax − HRrest) × .60 + HRrest
THR = (195 − 55) × .60 + 55
THR (lower) = (140) × .60 + 55
THR (lower) = 84 + 55
THR (lower) = 139 bt/min

Step 2: Calculate upper bound.

THR (upper) = (HR max − HRrest) × .80 + HRrest
= (195 − 55) × .80 + 55
= (140) (.8) + 55
= 112 + 55
= 167 bt/min

Mr. Jones' THR should be between 139 and 167 bt/min.

When a GXT is not performed, a THR can still be calculated using a maximum heart rate based on 220 minus age. In Example 6K the estimated maximum heart rate for Mr. Jones would be 220 − 30 = 190 bt/min. According to the Karvonen formula his THR range would be:

THR (lower bound) = (190 − 55) × .60 + 55
= (135) × .60 + 55
= 136 bt/min
THR (upper bound) = (190 − 55) .80 + 55
= (135) × .80 + 55
= 163 bt/min

Mr. Jones' training heart rate based on an estimated maximum HR would be 136–163 bt/min.

Summary of Training Heart Rate

Training heart rate should be viewed as nothing more than a guide to proper exercise intensity. The estimation of HRmax based on age has an error of around plus or minus 12 bt/min. Factors such as effort perception, medication, health and exercise history, motivation, exercise mode, climate, and altitude will affect the intensity of effort and HR response to exercise and need to be considered in the exercise prescription.

Summary

The calculations you worked with in this chapter are used frequently in the exercise lab and also in less formal exercise settings such as gyms or fitness centers. Calculating resting energy expenditure, converting METS to kcals, and using the Karvonen formula are integral to the work of an exercise professional. These calculations as well as material pertaining to specificity, sensitivity, and the Bayes theorem will be found on examinations for national certification and on exercise physiology college exams.

The following practice problems proceed from basic to complex. Completion of these calculations will help you feel comfortable and more familiar with all of the topics, numbers, and values in this chapter.

Chapter 6 Practice Problems

1. Use the Harris-Benedict equation to determine REE on these men. Round off each answer to the nearest kcal.

	Weight	Height	Age
(a)	95 kg	190 cm	40
(b)	75 kg	170 cm	40

2. A man and a woman both are 30 years old, weigh 140 lb, and are 68 in tall. Both are healthy but sedentary. Calculate REE for the two subjects. Which has the higher REE? When doing REE calculations only, round off the answer.

3. A female subject, 35 years old, is 63 in tall and weighs 140 lb. What is her REE for 1 hr?

4. A subject exercises at a 12-MET level for 45 min. How many kcal are expended? Use 1 MET = 1 kcal/kg/hr as the conversion factor. Subject's wt is 94 kg.

5. A subject exercises for 25 min at a 9-MET level and for another 35 min at a 12-MET level. This workout is performed three times per week. How many kcal are expended in 1 week? Subject weighs 68 kg.

   Hint: Use $\frac{1 \text{ kcal/kg/hr}}{1 \text{ MET}}$ as the conversion factor.

6. How many kcals are expended in 95 min of exercise at a 14-MET level? Subject weighs 72 kg. (Review example 6E.)

   Use $\frac{3.5 \text{ ml } O_2\text{/kg/min}}{1 \text{ MET}}$ as the conversion factor.

7. A man is exercising at a $\dot{V}O_2$ of $\frac{2{,}520 \text{ ml } O_2}{\text{min}}$.

   How many minutes of exercise will be needed to work off 1 lb of fat?

8. Barbara Ann, who weighs 65 kg, performs a workout of 10 METs for 15 min, 15 METS for 38 min, and 8 METS for 12 min. How many workouts will be required for her to expend 17,500 kcal?

   Use $\frac{3.5 \text{ ml } O_2/\text{kg}/\text{min}}{1 \text{ MET}}$ as the conversion factor. Use calculation method from Example 6E.

9. Determine the sensitivity of a GXT in a population of 43 patients with CAD, given 38 true positive GXTs and 5 false negative GXTs.

10. Determine the sensitivity of a GXT in a population of 985 patients with CAD, given 924 true positive GXTs and 61 false negative GXTs.

11. Determine the specificity of a GXT in a population of 62 apparently healthy individuals who walk for exercise, given 56 true negative GXTs and 6 false positive GXTs.

12. Determine the specificity of a GXT in a population of 895 apparently healthy runners, given 834 true negative GXTs and 61 false positive GXTs.

13. A 65-year-old female with non-anginal chest pain (chest pain after breakfast every day) performed a GXT. Pretest likelihood of heart disease was about 19% (Table 6.1). The test was negative for ST segment changes. Using the concept of Bayes theorem, which answer (a) or (b) would most closely represent this subject's posttest likelihood of heart disease? First, take an educated guess. Secondly, use Figure 6.1 to confirm your guess.

    (a) 10% or less likelihood of heart disease

    (b) 80% likelihood of heart disease

14. Harold, a 45-year-old steel worker, experiences typical jaw and chest anginal discomfort upon exertion, especially when walking up a hill. His pretest likelihood of CAD (Table 6.1) is 87.3%. The results of his GXT were positive for angina and showed significant ST segment depression.

    Use the concept of Bayes theorem to determine which of the percentages below would best represent this man's likelihood of heart disease after the GXT. First, take an educated guess. Secondly, confirm your answer using Figure 6.1.

    (a) 20% likelihood

    (b) 60% likelihood

    (c) 80% likelihood

    (d) 90–99% likelihood

15. Using Table 6.1, determine pretest likelihood of CAD for the following subjects.

    (a) Male, age 65, asymptomatic

    (b) Female, age 35, atypical angina

    (c) Typical angina, male, age 35

16. Use Bayes theorem to determine posttest probability of CAD in a 50-year-old male with atypical angina. His GXT was positive for 2 mm ST segment depression. Use the positive test equation.

Given sen = .70, spec = .90, and pretest likelihood (see Table 6.1),

$$\text{Posttest probability (pos)} = \frac{\text{pre} \times \text{sen}}{(\text{pre} \times \text{sen}) + (1 - \text{pre})(1 - \text{spec})}$$

17. Use Bayes theorem to calculate posttest probability of CAD in a male, age 65, whose GXT was negative for ST changes. Pretest symptoms were non-anginal chest pain. Sensitivity was .70 and specificity was .90.

18. Use the given information to determine posttest probability of CAD.

    Gender = male, age = 35, and symptoms = typical angina. The GXT ECG was positive for 2 mm ST segment depression. The sensitivity of GXT ECG in this population = 75% and specificity of GXT ECG in this population = 85%.

19. Determine posttest probability of CAD. Gender = female, age = 65, symptoms = atypical angina. The GXT ECG was negative for ST segment changes, sensitivity = .75, and specificity = .85.

20. Use the Karvonen formula to determine the THR. Use 60–80% of HRmax as the desired exercise intensity. Age = 35, weight = 76 kg, height = 72 in, HRmax = 184 bt/min, and resting HR = 64 bt/min.

21. A 20-year-old male has an exercise prescription for a THR of 80%–90% of his age-predicted HR. No stress test was performed. Using the Karvonen formula calculate his THR, given age = 20 and resting HR = 54.

Chapter 6 Answers to Practice Problems

1. REE

   (a) 2,053 kcal/24 hr

   (b) 1,678 kcal/24 hr

2. The male has a slightly higher REE.

   Male = 66.473 + 875.12726 + 864.11816 − 202.65 = 1,603 kcal/24 hr

   Female = 655.096 + 608.55453 + 319.532 − 140.28 = 1,443 kcal/24 hr

3. REE for an hour; female, age 35.

   Step 1: Convert lb to kg.

   $$140 \cancel{\text{lb}} \times \frac{1 \text{ kg}}{2.2 \cancel{\text{lb}}} = 64 \text{ kg}$$

   Step 2: Convert in to cm.

   $$63 \cancel{\text{in}} \times \frac{2.54 \text{ cm}}{1 \cancel{\text{in}}} = 160 \text{ cm}$$

   Step 3: Write out the Harris-Benedict equation.

   $$\text{Female} \frac{\text{kcal}}{24 \text{ hr}} = [655.096 + (9.563 \times \text{wt}) + (1.85 \times \text{ht})] - (4.676 \times \text{age})$$

$$\frac{1{,}399.468\text{ kcal}}{24\text{ hr}} = (655.096 + 612.032 + 296) - 163.66$$

REE = approx. 1,400 kcal/24 hr

Step 4: Convert kcal/24 hr to kcal/hr.

$$\frac{1{,}400\text{ kcal}}{24\text{ hr}} = \frac{58.33\text{ kcal}}{1\text{ hr}}\text{ rounded to 58 kcal/hr}$$

4. At a 12-MET level of exercise, 846 kcal will be consumed in 45 min.

Step 1: Convert METs to kcal/kg/hr

$$12\text{ }\cancel{\text{METs}} \times \frac{1\text{ kcal/kg/hr}}{1\text{ }\cancel{\text{MET}}} = 12\text{ kcal/kg/hr}$$

Step 2: Convert kcal/kg/hr to kcal/hr

$$\frac{12\text{ kcal}}{\cancel{\text{kg}}\text{/hr}} \times 94\text{ }\cancel{\text{kg}} = \frac{1{,}128\text{ kcal}}{\text{hr}}\text{ or }\frac{1{,}128\text{ kcal}}{60\text{ min}}$$

Step 3: Convert kcal/60 min to kcal expended in 45 min.

$$\frac{1{,}128\text{ kcal}}{60\text{ }\cancel{\text{min}}} \times 45\text{ }\cancel{\text{min}} = 846\text{ kcal}$$

5. Number of kcal expended in three workouts. (Review Example 6C).

Step 1: 9 METs for 25 min = 255 kcal

Step 2: 12 METs for 35 min = + 476 kcal

731 kcal/workout

$$\text{Step 3: }\frac{3\text{ }\cancel{\text{workouts}}}{1\text{ week}} \times \frac{731\text{ kcal}}{\cancel{\text{workout}}} = \frac{2{,}193\text{ kcal consumed}}{\text{week}}$$

6. In 95 min at 14 METS, 1,675.8 kcal will be expended. (Review example 6E.)

$$\text{Conversion factor: }\frac{3.5\text{ ml }O_2\text{/kg/min}}{1\text{ MET}}$$

Step 1: Convert METs to ml O_2/kg/min.

$$14\text{ }\cancel{\text{METs}} \times \frac{3.5\text{ ml }O_2\text{/kg/min}}{\cancel{\text{MET}}} = 49\text{ ml }O_2\text{/kg/min}$$

Step 2: Convert the relative $\dot{V}O_2$ to an absolute $\dot{V}O_2$.

(Relative $\dot{V}O_2$) (Absolute $\dot{V}O_2$)

$$\frac{49\text{ ml }O_2}{\cancel{\text{kg}}\text{/min}} \times 72\text{ }\cancel{\text{kg}} = \frac{3{,}528\text{ ml }O_2}{\text{min}}$$

Step 3: Convert absolute $\dot{V}O_2$ to kcal/min.

$$\frac{3{,}528\text{ }\cancel{\text{ml }O_2}}{\text{min}} \times \frac{.005\text{ kcal}}{\cancel{\text{ml }O_2}} = \frac{17.64\text{ kcal}}{\text{min}}$$

Step 4: Convert the kcal/min to kcal expended in 95 min.

$$\frac{17.64 \text{ kcal}}{\cancel{\text{min}}} \times \frac{95 \cancel{\text{min}}}{\text{one workout}} = \frac{1{,}675.8 \text{ kcal}}{\text{one workout}}$$

7. Minutes to expend 1 lb of fat. Conversion factor $\frac{3{,}500 \text{ kcal}}{1 \text{ lb fat}}$

Step 1: Convert the absolute $\dot{V}O_2$ to kcal/min.

$$\frac{2{,}520 \cancel{\text{ml } O_2}}{\text{min}} \times \frac{.005 \text{ kcal}}{\cancel{\text{ml } O_2}} = \frac{12.6 \text{ kcal}}{1 \text{ min}}$$

Step 2: Convert min/kcal to min to expend 1 lb of fat.

$$\frac{3{,}500 \cancel{\text{kcal}}}{1 \text{ lb fat}} \times \frac{1 \text{ min}}{12.6 \cancel{\text{kcal}}} = \frac{278 \text{ min}}{1 \text{ lb fat}}$$

This step can also be expressed as follows:

$$\frac{1 \text{ lb fat}}{3{,}500 \cancel{\text{kcal}}} \times \frac{12.6 \cancel{\text{kcal}}}{1 \text{ min}} = \frac{1 \text{ lb fat}}{278 \text{ min}}$$

Step 3: One pound of body fat is expended in 278 min (4.6 hr) while working at a $\dot{V}O_2$ of 2,520 ml O_2/min.

8. Workouts to expend 17,500 kcal (5 lb of body fat)

Step 1: Convert METs to ml O_2/kg/min.

Step 2: Convert ml O_2/kg/min to ml O_2/min.

Step 3: Convert ml O_2/min to kcal/min.

Step 4: Convert kcal/min to kcal.

$$\frac{11.375 \text{ kcal}}{\cancel{\text{min}}} \times 15 \cancel{\text{min}} = 170.625 \text{ kcal}$$
$$\frac{17.0625 \text{ kcal}}{\cancel{\text{min}}} \times 38 \cancel{\text{min}} = 648.375 \text{ kcal}$$
$$\frac{9.1 \text{ kcal}}{\cancel{\text{min}}} \times 12 \cancel{\text{min}} = +109.200 \text{ kcal}$$
$$928.2 \text{ kcal/workout}$$

Step 5: Convert kcal/workout to workouts.

$$\frac{17{,}500 \cancel{\text{kcal}}}{\text{to use 5 lb}} \times \frac{\text{workout}}{928.2 \cancel{\text{kcal}}} = \frac{19 \text{ workouts}}{\text{to use 5 lb}}$$

Step 6: Nineteen workouts are required to expend 5 lb of fat.

9. Sensitivity $= \frac{38}{38 + 5} \times 100\% = 88\%$

In this population the GXT correctly identified CAD 88% of the time.

10. Sensitivity $= \frac{924}{924 + 61} = \frac{924}{985} \times 100\% = 94\%$

In this population the GXT correctly identified CAD 94% of the time.

11. Specificity $= \frac{56}{56 + 6} \times 100\% = 90\%$

In this population the GXT correctly identified healthy subjects 90% of the time.

12. Specificity $= \dfrac{834}{834 + 61} \times 100\% = 93.2\%$

13. (a) 10% or less likelihood of CAD

14. (d) 90–99% likelihood of CAD

15. (a) 12.3%

    (b) 4.2%

    (c) 69.7%

16. Pre = 58.9%

$$\text{Posttest probability (pos)} = \frac{.589 \times .70}{(.589 \times .70) + (1 - .589)(1 - .90)}$$

$$\text{Posttest probability (pos)} = \frac{.4123}{.4534} = 91\% \text{ probability of CAD}$$

17. Pre = .281 (28.1%)

$$\text{Posttest probability (neg)} = \frac{.281 \times (1 - .70)}{.281 \times (1 - .70) + (1 - .281)(.90)}$$

$$\text{Posttest probability (neg)} = \frac{.0843}{.7314}$$

$$= 11.5\% \text{ probability of CAD}$$

18. Posttest probability of CAD would be 92%. The pretest = 69.7%.

    Compare this answer with Figure 6.1, where the sensitivity and specificity are the same as for this problem and problem 19.

19. Posttest probability of CAD in this female with her negative GXT would be 26%. Compare this answer with information in Figure 6.1.

20. Karvonen formula: 136 − 160 bt/min = THR

21. Karvonen formula

    Step 1: Determine predicted HRmax.

$$\begin{array}{r} 220 \\ -\ \ 20 \\ \hline 200 \end{array} - 54 = 146$$

    Step 2: Multiply 80% and 90% times the HRmax and add the resting HR back into the problem.

(Lower end of THR)	(Upper end of THR)
$146 \times .80 = 117$	$146 \times .90 = 131$
$+ 54$	$+ 54$
171	185

    Step 3: The THR is 171 − 185 bt/min.

7 Energy Cost of Level Walking

Major Concepts

Solving for $\dot{V}O_2$ using the level walking equation

Solving for walking speed when total $\dot{V}O_2$ is known

Determining average total $\dot{V}O_2$

This chapter and the next two chapters will show you how to estimate the energy costs of level walking, uphill walking, and running, respectively. You will learn how to work with the methods available for predicting these energy costs—methods often used in exercise prescription.

For calculations concerning all of these activities we will work with the ACSM metabolic equations for determining $\dot{V}O_2$ as listed in Appendix D. Each of these equations has its own constants ($\dot{V}O_2$ values), that is, built-in conversion factors derived from direct measurements of $\dot{V}O_2$ uptake during various types of exercises, to help us convert from the units that we are given to the units we want in our answer. The most notable of these constants, used as a standard in most of the ACSM equations, is the MET value you are already familiar with—3.5 ml O_2/kg/min = 1 MET.

Determining Total $\dot{V}O_2$ During Walking

Walking is defined as a gait in which the feet are lifted alternately with one foot not leaving the ground before the other foot touches down. The ACSM (1995) equations are most accurate for estimating $\dot{V}O_2$ with walking speeds between 1.9 mph (50 m/min) and 3.7 mph (100 m/min).

Solving for $\dot{V}O_2$ and METs

Total consumption of O_2 during walking is composed of two components, the energy required to move along level ground (horizontal component) and the energy required to move uphill (vertical component), plus the energy required to maintain resting metabolism.

The horizontal component is:

$$\dot{V}O_2 \text{ (ml/kg/min)} = \text{walking speed (m/min)} \times \frac{0.1 \text{ ml } O_2\text{/kg/min}}{\text{m/min}}$$

The vertical component is:

$$\dot{V}O_2 \text{ (ml/kg/min)} = \text{\% grade} \times \text{speed (m/min)} \times \frac{1.8 \text{ ml } O_2\text{/kg/min}}{\text{m/min}}$$

Resting $\dot{V}O_2$ is the other factor needed:

$$\text{Resting } \dot{V}O_2 = 3.5 \text{ ml } O_2\text{/kg/min (i.e., 1 MET)}$$

The constants represent the O_2 energy costs of the two types of walking. The $\dot{V}O_2$ constants are included in the equation so that m/min can be easily converted to ml O_2/kg/min. The constants

$$\dot{V}O_2 = \frac{0.1 \text{ ml } O_2\text{/kg/min}}{\text{m/min}}$$

and

$$\dot{V}O_2 = \frac{1.8 \text{ ml } O_2\text{/kg/min}}{\text{m/min}}$$

reflect the obvious difference in the energy cost of walking on level ground versus walking uphill. When you calculate the energy cost of level walking you ignore the vertical component.

The level walking equation is as follows:

$$\dot{V}O_2 \text{ walking on level (ml } O_2\text{/kg/min)} = \text{horizontal component} + \text{rest component}$$

$$\dot{V}O_2 \text{ walking on level (ml } O_2\text{/kg/min)} = \text{speed m/min} \times \frac{0.1 \text{ ml } O_2\text{/kg/min}}{\text{m/min}} + 3.5 \text{ ml } O_2\text{/kg/min}$$

Let's look at an example.

Example 7A

Determine total $\dot{V}O_2$ and MET level. Holly is walking on a level treadmill at 3 mph. Find her total $\dot{V}O_2$ and METs.

Step 1: Write out the formula.

$$\dot{V}O_2 \text{ (ml } O_2\text{/kg/min level)} = \text{speed (m/min)} \times \frac{.1 \text{ ml } O_2\text{/kg/min}}{\text{m/min}} + 3.5 \text{ ml } O_2\text{/kg/min}$$

Step 2: Because speed is given in mph, convert to m/min. Use the conversion factor 1 mph = 26.8 m/min. (See chapter 3 if you need to review this.)

$$3 \cancel{\text{mph}} \times \frac{26.8 \text{ m/min}}{1 \cancel{\text{mph}}} = 80.4 \text{ m/min}$$

Step 3: Plug the values into the formula and solve.

$$\dot{V}O_2 \text{ (ml } O_2\text{/kg/min level)} = \left(80.4 \cancel{\text{m/min}} \times \frac{0.1 \text{ ml } O_2\text{/kg/min}}{\cancel{\text{m/min}}}\right) + 3.5 \text{ ml } O_2\text{/kg/min}$$

$$\dot{V}O_2 \text{ (ml } O_2\text{/kg/min level)} = \left(80.4 \times 0.1 \text{ ml } O_2\text{/kg/min}\right) + 3.5 \text{ ml } O_2\text{/kg/min}$$

$$\dot{V}O_2 \text{ (ml } O_2\text{/kg/min)} = 11.54$$

Step 4: Convert to METs; use 1 MET = 3.5 ml O_2/kg/min.

$$11.54 \cancel{\text{ml } O_2\text{/kg/min}} \times \frac{1 \text{ MET}}{3.5 \cancel{\text{ml } O_2\text{/kg/min}}} = 3.30 \text{ METs}$$

Therefore, while Holly walks on a level TM at 3 mph (80.4 m/min), a comfortable walking speed, her total $\dot{V}O_2$ is 11.54 ml O_2/kg/min or 3.30 METs, a little over three times her resting metabolic rate. Don't forget to add the resting component when using the prediction equations to estimate total O_2 consumption during exercise. Avoid this very common error!

Solving for Walking Speed to Approximate a Given Energy Cost

In some cases, such as in exercise prescription, it is necessary to find the approximate walking speed that will elicit a desired level of oxygen consumption. This can be done by rearranging the equation for the total $\dot{V}O_2$ as follows.

$$\text{Total } \dot{V}O_2 \text{ (level walk ml } O_2\text{/kg/min)} = \left(\text{speed m/min} \times \frac{0.1 \text{ ml } O_2\text{/kg/min}}{\text{m/min}}\right) + 3.5 \text{ ml } O_2\text{/kg/min}$$

The goal is to isolate speed on one side of the equation. (See chapter 2 for review.) First subtract 3.5 ml O_2/kg/min from both sides:

$$\text{Total } \dot{V}O_2 \text{ (ml } O_2\text{/kg/min)} - 3.5 \text{ ml/kg/min} = \text{speed m/min} \times \frac{0.1 \text{ ml } O_2\text{/kg/min}}{\text{m/min}}$$

Dividing both sides by 0.1 ml O_2/kg/min will isolate speed (same as multiplying by 1 over .1 ml/kg/min):

$$\frac{\text{m/min (Total } \dot{V}O_2 \text{ (ml } O_2\text{/kg/min)} - 3.5 \text{ ml } O_2\text{/kg/min)}}{0.1 \text{ ml/kg/min}} = \text{speed}$$

$$\text{So Speed (m/min)} = \frac{\text{total } \dot{V}O_2 \text{ (ml } O_2\text{/kg/min)} - 3.5 \text{ ml } O_2\text{/kg/min}}{0.1 \text{ ml } O_2\text{/kg/min}}$$

The next example illustrates this calculation.

Example 7B

Solve for speed. Mr. Walker is asked to walk at a speed that would require a total $\dot{V}O_2$ of 13 ml O_2/kg/min. Because of a low-back problem he must walk on a level surface. At what speed should he walk?

Step 1: Use the formula for speed.

$$\text{Speed (m/min)} = \frac{\text{total } \dot{V}O_2 \text{ (ml } O_2\text{/kg/min)} - 3.5 \text{ ml } O_2\text{/kg/min}}{0.1 \text{ ml } O_2\text{/kg/min}}$$

$$\text{Speed} = \frac{13.0 - 3.5}{.1}$$

$$\text{Speed} = 95 \text{ m/min}$$

Or we could convert to miles per hour using the conversion factor 1 mph = 26.8 m/min:

$$95 \text{ m/min} \times \frac{1 \text{ mph}}{26.8 \text{ m/min}} = 3.54 \text{ mph}$$

So if Mr. Walker walks at about 3.5 mph on a level treadmill or around a level track he will meet the exercise prescription of 13 ml O_2/kg/min.

Using the Level Walking Equation to Determine Average Total $\dot{V}O_2$

We will now consider an assessment procedure that is a practical application of the level walking equation: determining steady-state $\dot{V}O_2$ during a 1.5-mile walk.

When the level walking equation is used in field testing for determining average total $\dot{V}O_2$, two tests are usually performed, one before and one after a period of fitness training. The only additional calculation needed for this assessment is initial conversion of the distance walked within a time period into a mph value. Two factors are required: the distance that is walked in feet or miles, usually 1 or 1.5 miles on a level walking surface, and the time period required for a subject to walk the measured distance.

Example 7C shows you how to calculate relative total $\dot{V}O_2$ for level walking.

Example 7C

Determine relative $\dot{V}O_2$ after a walking test. Roxanne has walked the testing distance of 7,920 ft within 30 min. Determine relative total $\dot{V}O_2$.

Step 1: Convert 7,920 ft/30 min into the unit miles/30 min. The conversion factor is 1 mile = 5,280 ft.

$$\frac{7{,}920 \text{ ft}}{30 \text{ min}} \times \frac{1 \text{ mile}}{5{,}280 \text{ ft}} = \frac{1.5 \text{ mile}}{30 \text{ min}}$$

Step 2: Convert the 1.5 mile/30 min into mph.

$$\frac{1.5 \text{ mile}}{30 \text{ min}} \times \frac{60 \text{ min}}{1 \text{ hr}} = \frac{3 \text{ mile}}{\text{hr}} \text{ or 3 mph}$$

Step 3: You can now plug the 3 mph (after converting to m/min) into the level walking equation to calculate the average total $\dot{V}O_2$ for that 1.5-mile distance.

Summary

This chapter has provided you with a straightforward approach for determining total $\dot{V}O_2$ using the equation for level walking, and for finding the speed of level walking when the total $\dot{V}O_2$ is known.

The practice problems that follow are ordered to progress from basic to more complex. By the time you complete the practice problems you will feel confident when presented with level walking problems on exams or in the field. You will also be prepared for the calculations involving percent grade treadmill walking in the next chapter. There we will add a third factor, treadmill elevation, which is the vertical $\dot{V}O_2$ component in the walking equation.

Chapter 7 Practice Problems

1. Convert the following walking speeds from mph to m/min.

   (a) 3.7 mph

   (b) 3.0 mph

2. Convert to mph.

   (a) 52 m/min

   (b) 62 m/min

3. Tracey is walking at a speed of 92 m/min. Find her total $\dot{V}O_2$.

   $$\text{Hint: Total } \dot{V}O_2 = \left(\text{speed} \times \frac{0.1 \text{ ml } O_2/\text{kg/min}}{\text{m/min}}\right) + 3.5 \text{ ml } O_2/\text{kg/min}$$

   $$\begin{aligned} \text{Horiz } \dot{V}O_2 &= \quad ? \text{ ml } O_2/\text{kg/min} \\ \text{Rest } \dot{V}O_2 &= \underline{+\ 3.5 \text{ ml } O_2/\text{kg/min}} \\ \text{Total } \dot{V}O_2 &= \quad ? \end{aligned}$$

4. Brenda is walking at a speed of 99 m/min on a level surface.

   Find her total $\dot{V}O_2$.

5. Convert these to ml O_2/min.

   (a) 2.5 L O_2 min^{-1}

   (b) $\frac{3.2 \text{ L } O_2}{\text{min}}$

6. Convert to $\frac{\text{L } O_2}{\text{min}}$. Round off your answer to two decimal places.

   (a) $3{,}600 \frac{\text{ml } O_2}{\text{min}}$

(b) $5{,}214 \frac{\text{ml } O_2}{\text{min}}$

(c) $2{,}790.345 \frac{\text{ml } O_2}{\text{min}}$

7. Given speed = 88 m/min, find total relative $\dot{V}O_2$.
8. Given speed = 2.8 mph, find total relative $\dot{V}O_2$ and METs.
9. Given total $\dot{V}O_2$ = 13.0 ml O_2/kg/min, find speed in m/min.

   (Remember to first subtract the resting $\dot{V}O_2$.)
10. Given total $\dot{V}O_2$ = 13.45 ml O_2/kg/min, find speed in m/min.
11. MET level = 3.4 METs; find m/min and mph.

    Hint: $3.4 \text{ METs} \times \frac{3.5 \text{ ml } O_2/\text{kg}/\text{min}}{1 \text{ MET}} = ?$
12. Given 2.8 METs, find m/min and mph.
13. Given total $\dot{V}O_2$ = 1.2 L O_2 min^{-1} and subject's weight = 100 kg, find speed.
14. Given $\dot{V}O_2$ = 0.56 L O_2 min^{-1} and weight = 70 kg, find speed.
15. Given total $\dot{V}O_2$ = 9.97 ml O_2/kg/min and horiz $\dot{V}O_2$ = 6.47 ml O_2/kg/min, find resting $\dot{V}O_2$.
16. Given speed = 100 m/min, find total $\dot{V}O_2$ and METs.
17. Given $\dot{V}O_2$ = 8.86 ml O_2/kg/min, find treadmill speed.
18. Kenneth, who weighs 72 kg, is walking at a speed of 3.6 mph. How many kcal will he expend during a 30-min walk on a level treadmill?

Chapter 7 Answers to Practice Problems

1. (a) $3.7 \cancel{\text{mph}} \times \frac{26.8 \text{ m/min}}{1 \cancel{\text{mph}}} = 99.16 \text{ m/min}$

   (b) 80.4 m/min

2. (a) $52 \cancel{\text{m/min}} \times \frac{1 \text{ mph}}{26.8 \cancel{\text{m/min}}} = 1.94 \text{ mph}$

   (b) 2.31 mph

3.
$$\begin{aligned} \text{Horiz } \dot{V}O_2 &= \quad 9.20 \text{ ml } O_2/\text{kg/min} \\ \text{Rest } \dot{V}O_2 &= + \ \underline{3.50 \text{ ml } O_2/\text{kg/min}} \\ & \quad\ 12.70 \text{ ml } O_2/\text{kg/min} = \text{total } \dot{V}O_2 \end{aligned}$$

4.
$$\begin{aligned} \text{Horiz } \dot{V}O_2 &= \quad 99.0 \cancel{\text{m/min}} \times \frac{0.1 \text{ ml } O_2/\text{kg/min}}{\cancel{\text{m/min}}} \\ \text{Horiz } \dot{V}O_2 &= \quad 9.90 \text{ ml } O_2/\text{kg/min} \\ \text{Rest } \dot{V}O_2 &= + \ \underline{3.50 \text{ ml } O_2/\text{kg/min}} \\ & \quad\ 13.40 \text{ ml } O_2/\text{kg/min} = \text{total } \dot{V}O_2 \end{aligned}$$

5. (a) $2.5 \text{ L } O_2 \text{ min}^{-1} = \frac{2{,}500 \text{ ml } O_2}{\text{min}}$

(b) $\frac{3.2 \text{ L } O_2}{\text{min}} = \frac{3{,}200 \text{ ml } O_2}{\text{min}}$

6. (a) $\frac{3.60 \text{ L } O_2}{\text{min}}$

(b) $5.21 \text{ L } O_2 \text{ min}^{-1}$ or $\frac{5.21 \text{ L } O_2}{\text{min}}$

(c) 2.79 L O_2/min

7. 12.30 ml O_2/kg/min (relative $\dot{V}O_2$)

8. 11.00 ml O_2/kg/min and 3.14 METs

9.
$$\begin{array}{rl} 13.0 \text{ ml } O_2/\text{kg/min} & = \text{total } \dot{V}O_2 \\ -\ 3.5 \text{ ml } O_2/\text{kg/min} & = \text{rest } \dot{V}O_2 \\ \hline 9.5 \text{ ml } O_2/\text{kg/min} & = \text{horiz } \dot{V}O_2 \end{array}$$

$$9.5 \cancel{\text{ml } O_2/\text{kg/min}} \times \frac{\text{m/min}}{0.1 \cancel{\text{ml } O_2/\text{kg/min}}} = 95 \text{ m/min (3.54 mph)}$$

10. Speed = 99.50 m/min

Note: Values greater than 13.50 ml O_2/kg/min for level walking are greater than the max defined walking speed of about 100 m/min or 3.7 mph (ACSM, 1995).

11. Speed = 84 m/min = 3.13 mph (11.9 ml O_2/kg/min = total $\dot{V}O_2$)

12. Speed = 63 m/min = 2.35 mph

13. $1.2 \text{ L min}^{-1} = 1{,}200 \text{ ml } O_2$

Total $\dot{V}O_2$ = 12 ml O_2/kg/min

Speed = 85 m/min (3.17 mph)

14. $\frac{0.56 \cancel{\text{L}}\ O_2}{\text{min}} \times \frac{1{,}000 \text{ ml}}{1 \cancel{\text{L}}} = \frac{560 \text{ ml } O_2}{\text{min}}$

$$\frac{560 \text{ ml } O_2/\text{min}}{70 \text{ kg}} = 8.0 \text{ ml } O_2/\text{kg/min (relative } \dot{V}O_2)$$

$$\begin{array}{rl} 8.0 \text{ ml } O_2/\text{kg/min} & = \text{total } \dot{V}O_2 \\ -\ 3.5 \text{ ml } O_2/\text{kg/min} & = \text{rest } \dot{V}O_2 \\ \hline 4.5 \text{ ml } O_2/\text{kg/min} & = \text{horiz } \dot{V}O_2 \end{array}$$

$$4.5 \cancel{\text{ml } O_2/\text{kg/min}} \times \frac{\text{m/min}}{0.1 \cancel{\text{ml } O_2/\text{kg/min}}} = 45 \text{ m/min} = \text{speed (1.68 mph)}$$

15. Rest $\dot{V}O_2$ = 3.5 ml O_2/kg/min. With all calculations, resting $\dot{V}O_2$ will always be the average value, 3.5 ml O_2/kg/min, unless it has been directly measured using open-circuit spirometry. In a very well conditioned athlete, resting $\dot{V}O_2$ may be 3.6 to 3.8 ml O_2/kg/min. In a very sedentary individual with low percentage of muscle mass and a high percentage of body fat, resting $\dot{V}O_2$ may range well below the 3.5 ml O_2/kg/min, to values such as 3.0 to 3.4 ml O_2/kg/min.

16. 13.50 ml O_2/kg/min and 3.86 METs
17. 53.6 m/min = 2 mph
18. Speed = 96.48 m/min

    Total $\dot{V}O_2$ = 13.148 ml O_2/kg/min (relative)

    Total $\dot{V}O_2$ = 946.656 ml O_2/min (absolute)

    kcal expenditure = 4.73328 kcal/min

    kcal expenditure = 141.9984 kcal, or about 142 kcal in 30 min

At this point you should be able to perform the level walking metabolic calculations easily. In the next chapter, percent grade will be added to the treadmill walking calculations.

8 Energy Cost of Uphill Walking

Major Concepts

Percent grade on a treadmill

The treadmill walking equation

Solving for $\dot{V}O_2$, walking speed and percent grade

As we saw in the last chapter, the horizontal and resting $\dot{V}O_2$ components are required to calculate a subject's total $\dot{V}O_2$ during level walking. In this chapter we will examine the equation used to calculate total $\dot{V}O_2$ when a subject is walking up an incline.

This information will help you prepare for the running math problems that are presented in chapter 9. Before investigating the inclined walking equation we will briefly consider the concept of percent grade.

Percent Grade on an Inclined Treadmill

To estimate the total $\dot{V}O_2$ of uphill walking the vertical energy cost component, which considers the steepness of the hill, must be included.

Most treadmills allow for adjustment of speed and elevation. The elevation is typically expressed as a percent grade. Percent grade is the preferred measure of elevation as opposed to angular degrees because percent grade allows for smaller increments of measure than degrees. A comparison of degrees and percent grade is shown in Table 8.1. A 2% grade is approximately a 1.15° angle, while a 1% grade represents a .575° angle above horizontal (0% grade).

The two most popular treadmill GXT protocols, the Balke (1959) and the Bruce (1973), are described in Table 8.2. You will find this table helpful to refer to as you read through the examples and perform the practice problems in this chapter.

Table 8.1 Comparison of % Grade and Degrees of an Angle

% Grade on a TM	=	Degrees of an angle
1		0.575
2		1.15
3		1.73
4		2.30
5		2.88
6		3.45
7		4.00
8		4.60
9		5.18
10		5.57
11		6.33
12		6.90
13		7.48
14		8.05
15		8.63
16		9.20
17		9.78
18		10.35
19		10.93
20		11.50

Treadmill Walking Equation: Level and Uphill

To calculate total $\dot{V}O_2$ for walking on a level surface or level treadmill, only the horizontal and resting $\dot{V}O_2$ are required, as we saw in chapter 7.

To make the walking equation complete, so that we can solve for total $\dot{V}O_2$ during walking up a percent grade, a vertical $\dot{V}O_2$ component must be added:

$$\text{Total } \dot{V}O_2 = (\text{horiz } \dot{V}O_2) + (\text{vert } \dot{V}O_2) + (\text{rest } \dot{V}O_2)$$

Calculation of the Vertical Component

The vertical component of total $\dot{V}O_2$ is calculated as follows:

$$\dot{V}O_2 \text{ (vertical ml } O_2\text{/kg/min)} = \text{\% grade} \times \text{speed (m/min)} \times \frac{1.8 \text{ ml } O_2\text{/kg/min}}{\text{m/min}}$$

The percent grade must be included as a decimal. For example, a 12% grade would be written .12, a 20% grade as .20, and so on. Speed must be in m/min. The constant

$$\frac{1.8 \text{ ml } O_2\text{/kg/min}}{\text{m/min}}$$

Table 8.2 Description of Balke and Bruce Graded Exercise Testing Protocols

Balke GXT protocol				Bruce GXT protocol			
Stage	min/stage	Speed (mph)	% grade	Stage	min/stage	Speed (mph)	% grade
1	1	3.3	0	1	3	1.7	10
2	1	3.3	2	2	3	2.5	12
3	1	3.3	3	3	3	3.4	14
4	1	3.3	4	4	3	4.2	16
5	1	3.3	5	5	3	5.0	18
6	1	3.3	6	6	3	5.5	20
7	1	3.3	7	7	3	6.0	22
8	1	3.3	8				
9	1	3.3	9				
10*	1	3.3	10				
—	—	—	—				
24	1	3.3	23				
25	1	3.4	23				
26	1	3.5	23				
27	1	3.6	23				
28	1	3.7	23				
29	1	3.8	23				

*The Balke continues adding 1% grade each min (stage) until the 24th minute. At this point the % grade remains at 23% and the speed increases by 0.1 mph each minute until the client fatigues or symptoms arise.

represents the O_2 cost of walking up an incline. Example 8A illustrates the calculation of the vertical component only, during walking at 53 m/min up an 8% grade. In Example 8B we will calculate the percent grade.

Example 8A

Find the vertical component of the total $\dot{V}O_2$. Jamie is walking on a treadmill at a speed of 53 m/min on an 8% grade. Find $\dot{V}O_2$ vertical.

Step 1: Speed is already in the correct units, m/min.

Step 2: Insert the known values into the vertical $\dot{V}O_2$ component. Perform the math.

$$\text{Vertical } \dot{V}O_2 = .08 \times 53 \text{ m/min} \times 1.8 \text{ ml } O_2\text{/kg/min}$$
$$\text{Vertical } \dot{V}O_2 = 7.632 \text{ ml } O_2\text{/kg/min}$$

If we did not know the percent grade but knew that the vertical component for $\dot{V}O_2$ was 7.632 ml O_2/kg/min at 53 m/min, we could then calculate the percent grade. The answer should be 8% as in Example 8A. Let's see whether it is.

Example 8B

Find percent grade. The vertical $\dot{V}O_2$ component and the speed are both known from Example 8A. Determine percent grade of the treadmill. This will provide a "proof" that the answer for Example 8A is correct.

Step 1: Write out the formula.

$$\text{Vertical } \dot{V}O_2 = \%\text{ grade} \times \text{speed m/min} \times \frac{1.8 \text{ ml } O_2/\text{kg/min}}{\text{m/min}}$$

Step 2: Plug in the known values.

$$7.632 \text{ ml } O_2/\text{kg/min} = \%\text{ grade} \times 53 \cancel{\text{m/min}} \times \frac{1.8 \text{ ml } O_2/\text{kg/min}}{\cancel{\text{m/min}}}$$

$$7.632 \text{ ml } O_2/\text{kg/min} = \%\text{ grade} \times 95.4 \text{ ml } O_2/\text{kg/min}$$

Step 3: Now, solve for the unknown % grade. Isolate the % grade to the right side of the equation. Divide both sides of the equation by the 95.4 ml O_2/kg/min. Use your pencil to cancel the like factors on the right side of the equation.

$$\frac{7.632 \text{ ml } O_2/\text{kg/min}}{95.4 \text{ ml } O_2/\text{kg/min}} = \%\text{ grade} \times \frac{95.4 \text{ ml } O_2/\text{kg/min}}{95.4 \text{ ml } O_2/\text{kg/min}}$$

Step 4: After the cancellation process, we are left with:

$$\frac{7.632 \cancel{\text{ml } O_2/\text{kg/min}}}{95.4 \cancel{\text{ml } O_2/\text{kg/min}}} = .08 = 8\%\text{ grade}$$

This agrees with the value given in Example 8A.

Setting Up the Walking Equation for Easy Calculation

Stacking the components and setting up the equation like an addition problem allows you to add numbers with decimals more easily and also to inspect the units to verify that they are all the same.

In this walking equation as well as the running equation in chapter 9, all of the numbers that are added together must have the unit ml O_2/kg/min. Like terms, or in this case, *like units,* can be added together:

$$\begin{aligned} \text{Horiz } \dot{V}O_2 &= 7.3 \text{ ml } O_2/\text{kg/min} \\ \text{Vert } \dot{V}O_2 &= 15.4 \text{ ml } O_2/\text{kg/min} \\ +\text{ Rest } \dot{V}O_2 &= 3.5 \text{ ml } O_2/\text{kg/min} \\ \hline \text{Total } \dot{V}O_2 &= 26.2 \text{ ml } O_2/\text{kg/min} \end{aligned}$$

As mentioned in the previous chapter, the most common error in performing the walking, running, cycle, or arm crank equations is the failure to add in the resting $\dot{V}O_2$ component.

Calculating Total $\dot{V}O_2$ During Graded Walking

The total $\dot{V}O_2$ is given by the equation in the ACSM *Guidelines For Exercise Testing And Prescription* (1995):

Total $\dot{V}O_2$ =

$$\left(\text{m/min} \times \frac{.01 \text{ ml } O_2/\text{kg/min}}{\text{m/min}}\right) + \left(\% \text{ grade} \times \text{m/min} \times \frac{1.8 \text{ ml } O_2/\text{kg/min}}{\text{m/min}}\right) + (3.5 \text{ ml } O_2/\text{kg/min})$$

(Horiz $\dot{V}O_2$) + (Vert $\dot{V}O_2$) + (Rest $\dot{V}O_2$)

This equation can be used to calculate total $\dot{V}O_2$ (ml O_2/kg/min), walking speed (m/min), or percent grade. Let's practice.

Example 8C

Calculate total oxygen consumption. Kevin is in stage 2 of the Bruce protocol (Table 8.2). His speed is 67 m/min and the grade is 12%. Find his total $\dot{V}O_2$ and METs.

Step 1: Calculate the horizontal $\dot{V}O_2$.

$$\text{Horiz } \dot{V}O_2 = 67 \cancel{\text{m/min}} \times \frac{0.1 \text{ ml } O_2/\text{kg/min}}{\cancel{\text{m/min}}} = 6.700 \text{ ml } O_2/\text{kg/min}$$

Step 2: Calculate the vertical $\dot{V}O_2$.

$$\text{Vert } \dot{V}O_2 = .12 \times 67 \cancel{\text{m/min}} \times \frac{1.8 \text{ ml } O_2/\text{kg/min}}{\cancel{\text{m/min}}} = 14.472 \text{ ml } O_2/\text{kg/min}$$

Step 3: No other calculation is necessary. We just need to add the resting component:

Rest $\dot{V}O_2$ = 3.500 ml O_2/kg/min

Step 4: Add the three $\dot{V}O_2$ components together.

$$\begin{array}{rrl} \text{Horiz } \dot{V}O_2 = & 6.700 & \text{ml } O_2/\text{kg/min} \\ \text{Vert } \dot{V}O_2 = & 14.472 & \text{ml } O_2/\text{kg/min} \\ + \text{ Rest } \dot{V}O_2 = & 3.500 & \text{ml } O_2/\text{kg/min} \\ \hline & 24.672 & \text{ml } O_2/\text{kg/min} \end{array}$$

= total relative $\dot{V}O_2$, rounded off to 24.67 ml O_2/kg/min

Step 5: Convert 24.67 ml O_2/kg/min to METs. Use your pencil to cancel the units.

$$24.67 \cancel{\text{ml } O_2/\text{kg/min}} \times \frac{1 \text{ MET}}{3.5 \cancel{\text{ml } O_2/\text{kg/min}}} = 7.05 \text{ METs}$$

Note that to achieve the best estimation of $\dot{V}O_2$ at any intensity of effort, a subject should walk or jog on the TM, if safety permits, without holding the handrail.

Example 8D

Find percent grade. The exercise prescription for Mr. Edwards states that he should walk at an intensity of about 7.2 METs. Because he has an artificial hip he cannot walk any faster than 50 m/min. He has no restriction on the amount of incline he can use. Given his walking speed, find the correct percent grade for the treadmill.

Step 1: Determine total $\dot{V}O_2$ from METs.

$$7.2\ \cancel{\text{METs}} \times \frac{3.5\text{ ml }O_2/\text{kg/min}}{1\ \cancel{\text{MET}}}$$
$$= 25.2\text{ ml }O_2/\text{kg/min, or approximately }25\text{ ml }O_2/\text{kg/min.}$$

Step 2: Subtract the rest $\dot{V}O_2$ from the total $\dot{V}O_2$.

$$\begin{array}{lr} \text{Total }\dot{V}O_2 = & 25.0\text{ ml }O_2/\text{kg/min} \\ \text{Rest }\dot{V}O_2 = & -\ 3.5\text{ ml }O_2/\text{kg/min} \\ \hline & 21.5\text{ ml }O_2/\text{kg/min} = \text{horiz }\dot{V}O_2 + \text{vert }\dot{V}O_2 \end{array}$$

Step 3: Find the horiz $\dot{V}O_2$. The 21.5 ml O_2/kg/min represents the combination of horizontal plus the vertical $\dot{V}O_2$. To find the vertical $\dot{V}O_2$ so that we can solve for percent grade, as we did in Example 8B, we must now find the horizontal $\dot{V}O_2$.

$$\text{Horiz }\dot{V}O_2 = \cancel{\text{m/min}} \times \frac{0.1\text{ ml }O_2/\text{kg/min}}{\cancel{\text{m/min}}}$$
$$\text{Horiz }\dot{V}O_2 = 50\text{ m/min} \times \frac{0.1\text{ ml }O_2/\text{kg/min}}{\text{m/min}}$$
$$\text{Horiz }\dot{V}O_2 = 5.0\text{ ml }O_2/\text{kg/min}$$

Step 4: Solve for vert $\dot{V}O_2$.
Subtract the horiz $\dot{V}O_2$ from the (horiz $\dot{V}O_2$ + vert $\dot{V}O_2$).

$$\begin{array}{rr} \text{Horiz }\dot{V}O_2 + \text{vert }\dot{V}O_2 = & 21.5\text{ ml }O_2/\text{kg/min} \\ \text{Horiz }\dot{V}O_2 = & -\ 5.0\text{ ml }O_2/\text{kg/min} \\ \hline & 16.5\text{ ml }O_2/\text{kg/min} = \text{vert }\dot{V}O_2 \end{array}$$

Step 5: Now that we have the value for the vert $\dot{V}O_2$, we must isolate the % grade. Write out the vertical $\dot{V}O_2$ equation.

$$\text{Vertical }\dot{V}O_2 = \left(\%\text{ grade} \times \text{m/min} \times \frac{1.8\text{ ml }O_2/\text{kg/min}}{\text{m/min}}\right)$$

Fill in the known values. Multiply m/min times the 1.8 constant.

$$16.5\text{ ml }O_2/\text{kg/min} = \left(\%\text{ grade} \times 50\ \cancel{\text{m/min}} \times \frac{1.8\text{ ml }O_2/\text{kg/min}}{\cancel{\text{m/min}}}\right)$$
$$16.5\text{ ml }O_2/\text{kg/min} = \%\text{ grade} \times 90\text{ ml }O_2/\text{kg/min}$$

Step 6: Isolate the % grade to the right side of the equation.

$$\frac{16.5 \text{ ml O}_2\text{/kg/min}}{90 \text{ ml O}_2\text{/kg/min}} = .183 = 18\% \text{ grade} \quad \text{(See Example 8B.)}$$

An 18% grade at 50 m/min yields a total $\dot{V}O_2$ of 25 ml O_2/kg/min, which is about 7.14 METs.

In Example 8E the exercise prescription requires the subject to walk at a 10% grade for leg strengthening at a $\dot{V}O_2$ of 35 ml O_2/kg/min. Determine the speed of the treadmill that will satisfy this $\dot{V}O_2$.

Example 8E

Determine treadmill speed when total $\dot{V}O_2$ is already known. Tracy is training on a treadmill at a 10% grade. Her total $\dot{V}O_2$ is 35 ml O_2/kg/min. Determine the correct walking speed for Tracy to train at.

Step 1: Write the equation.

$$\text{Total } \dot{V}O_2 = 35 \text{ ml O}_2\text{/kg/min} =$$

$$\left(\text{speed} \times \frac{0.1 \text{ m O}_2\text{/kg/min}}{\text{m/min}}\right) + \left(\text{speed} \times .10 \times \frac{1.8 \text{ ml O}_2\text{/kg/min}}{\text{m/min}}\right) + (3.5 \text{ ml O}_2\text{/kg/min})$$

Step 2: Subtract the rest $\dot{V}O_2$ from the total $\dot{V}O_2$.

$$\begin{aligned} \text{Total } \dot{V}O_2 &= \quad 35.0 \text{ ml O}_2\text{/kg/min} \\ \text{Rest } \dot{V}O_2 &= -\ \ 3.5 \text{ ml O}_2\text{/kg/min} \\ & \quad\ 31.5 \text{ ml O}_2\text{/kg/min} = \text{horiz } \dot{V}O_2 + \text{vert } \dot{V}O_2 \end{aligned}$$

Step 3: Rewrite the equation without the rest $\dot{V}O_2$. Cancel the m/min; then multiply .10 × 1.8.

$$(\text{Horiz } \dot{V}O_2) \qquad + (\text{Vert } \dot{V}O_2)$$

$$31.5 \text{ ml O}_2\text{/kg/min} = \left(\text{speed} \times \frac{0.1 \text{ ml O}_2\text{/kg/min}}{\text{m/min}}\right) + \left(\text{speed} \times .10 \times \frac{1.8 \text{ ml O}_2\text{/kg/min}}{\text{m/min}}\right)$$

$$31.5 \text{ ml O}_2\text{/kg/min} = \left(\text{speed} \times \frac{0.1 \text{ ml O}_2\text{/kg/min}}{\text{m/min}}\right) + \left(\text{speed} \times \frac{0.18 \text{ ml O}_2\text{/kg/min}}{\text{m/min}}\right)$$

Check your math for this and the next two steps (S = speed):

$$\begin{aligned} 31.5 &= (S \times 0.1) + (S \times 0.18) \\ 31.5 &= S\,(0.1 + 0.18) \\ 31.5 &= S \times 0.28 \\ \frac{31.5}{0.28} &= 112.5 \text{ m/min} = S \end{aligned}$$

Step 4: Add like terms together.

$$0.1 \text{ ml O}_2\text{/kg/min} + 0.18 \text{ ml O}_2\text{/kg/min} = 0.28 \text{ ml O}_2\text{/kg/min}$$

The term *speed* is retained, not added together.

$$31.5 \text{ ml } O_2/\text{kg}/\text{min} = \text{speed} \times \frac{0.28 \text{ ml } O_2/\text{kg}/\text{min}}{\text{m}/\text{min}}$$

Step 5: Isolate speed on the right side of the equation. Invert the fraction and multiply. Cancel the ml O_2/kg/min.

$$31.5 \cancel{\text{ml } O_2/\text{kg}/\text{min}} \times \frac{\text{m}/\text{min}}{0.28 \cancel{\text{ml } O_2/\text{kg}/\text{min}}} = \text{speed}$$

$$112.5 \text{ m}/\text{min} = \text{speed}$$

Step 6: Convert the m/min to mph.

$$112.5 \cancel{\text{m}/\text{min}} \times \frac{\text{mph}}{26.8 \cancel{\text{m}/\text{min}}} = \text{about } 4.2 \text{ mph}$$

At a $\dot{V}O_2$ of 35 ml O_2/kg/min and a 10% grade on the TM, the walking speed is about 4.2 miles/hr.

Summary

In this chapter we discussed the method of determining total $\dot{V}O_2$ for walking on an inclined treadmill. The level walking equation and the equation for walking up an incline were compared. The inclined walking equation includes a vertical $\dot{V}O_2$ component.

We discussed rearranging the entire inclined walking equation to solve for percent grade or to solve for walking speed. Having learned to solve for percent grade and walking speed, as well as total $\dot{V}O_2$, you are now ready to progress to the practice problems for this chapter.

Chapter 8 Practice Problems

Round off final answers to two decimal places.

1. Convert the following to m/min.

   (a) 2 mph (b) 3.5 mph

2. Convert the following to mph.

   (a) 98 m/min (b) 67 m/min

3. Given 53 m/min, find horiz $\dot{V}O_2$.

4. Determine vertical $\dot{V}O_2$ only for each of the following.

   (a) 53 m/min and 6% grade

   (b) 3.5 mph and 8% grade

5. Mary Jean, who weighs 54 kg, is walking on a treadmill with a 6% grade at 92 m/min. Determine: total relative $\dot{V}O_2$, METs, total absolute $\dot{V}O_2$, and kcal expended per minute.

6. Determine treadmill walking speed given the following. Review example 8E if you need to.
   (a) Given total $\dot{V}O_2$ = 25 ml O_2/kg/min and grade = 9%
   (b) Given total $\dot{V}O_2$ = 2.448 L O_2/min, grade = 12%, and subject's wt = 72 kg
7. Determine percent grade for each of the following.
   (a) Given vert $\dot{V}O_2$ = 13 ml O_2/kg/min and speed = 80 m/min
   (b) Given vert $\dot{V}O_2$ = 12 ml O_2/kg/min and speed = 74 m/min
8. Mr. Smith is walking on a treadmill at a speed of 45 m/min at a 2% grade. How much oxygen is he consuming at this speed and grade and what is his MET level? Remember that speed is entered into the equation in two places.
9. Mr. Sherman is walking on a treadmill without holding on to the handrail at a speed of 3 mph with a grade of 4%. Determine total $\dot{V}O_2$.
10. Given total $\dot{V}O_2$ = 20.1 ml O_2/kg/min and speed = 68 m/min, find percent grade.
11. Given total $\dot{V}O_2$ = 28 ml O_2/kg/min and speed = 53 m/min, find percent grade.
12. Given total $\dot{V}O_2$ = 28 ml O_2/kg/min and grade = 9%, find speed.
13. Given total $\dot{V}O_2$ = 15 ml O_2/kg/min and grade = 2%, find speed.
14. Scotty, who weighs 176 lb, walked on a TM with a 10% grade at a speed of 100 m/min for 55 min. Determine the following.
    (a) Total relative $\dot{V}O_2$
    (b) MET level
    (c) Subject's weight in kg
    (d) Total absolute $\dot{V}O_2$
    (e) kcal expended per minute
    (f) kcal expended in the 55 min

Answers to Chapter 8 Practice Problems

1. (a) $2 \not{\text{mph}} \times \dfrac{26.8 \text{ m/min}}{1 \not{\text{mph}}} = 53.6 \text{ m/min}$

   (b) 93.8 m/min

2. (a) $98 \not{\text{m/min}} \times \dfrac{1 \text{ mph}}{26.8 \not{\text{m/min}}} = 3.66 \text{ mph}$

   (b) 2.5 mph

3. $\text{Horiz } \dot{V}O_2 = 53 \not{\text{m/min}} \times \dfrac{0.1 \text{ ml } O_2/\text{kg/min}}{\not{\text{m/min}}}$

   $\text{Horiz } \dot{V}O_2 = 5.3 \text{ ml } O_2/\text{kg/min}$

4. (a) Vert $\dot{V}O_2 = .06 \times 53\ \cancel{m/min} \times \frac{1.8\ ml\ O_2/kg/min}{\cancel{m/min}}$

   Vert $\dot{V}O_2 = 5.72\ ml\ O_2/kg/min$

   (b) $13.51\ ml\ O_2/kg/min$

5. Total $\dot{V}O_2 = 22.636\ ml\ O_2/kg/min$, 6.47 METs

$$\frac{1222.344\ \cancel{ml\ O_2}}{min} \times \frac{.005\ kcal}{\cancel{ml\ O_2}} = \text{approx}\ \frac{6.11\ kcal}{min}$$

6. Given total $\dot{V}O_2$, find speed.

   (a) Step 1: Subtract resting $\dot{V}O_2$.

$$\begin{array}{lrl} \text{Total } \dot{V}O_2 = & & 25.0\ ml\ O_2/kg/min \\ \text{Rest } \dot{V}O_2 = & - & 3.5\ ml\ O_2/kg/min \\ \hline & & 21.5\ ml\ O_2/kg/min = \text{horiz} + \text{vert } \dot{V}O_2 \end{array}$$

   Step 2: Math check: Add like terms.

   $0.1 + (.09 \times 1.8) = .262$

   Step 3: Isolate speed.

$$21.5\ \cancel{ml\ O_2/kg/min} \times \frac{m/min}{.262\ \cancel{ml\ O_2/kg/min}} = \text{speed}$$

$$82.06\ m/min = \text{speed}$$

   (b) Total $\dot{V}O_2$ (relative) $= 34\ ml\ O_2/kg/min$

   Math check: $\frac{30.5}{.316} = 96.52\ m/min$ (approx. 3.6 mph)

7. (a) $13\ ml\ O_2/kg/min = ?\ \text{grade} \times 80\ \cancel{m/min} \times \frac{1.8\ ml\ O_2/kg/min}{\cancel{m/min}}$

$$\frac{13\ \cancel{ml\ O_2/kg/min}}{144\ \cancel{ml\ O_2/kg/min}} = ?\ \text{grade}$$

   $.09 = \text{grade} = 9\%$

   (b) .09 or 9%

8. Total $\dot{V}O_2 = ?$

   Step 1: Find horiz $\dot{V}O_2$.

$$\text{Horiz } \dot{V}O_2 = 45\ \cancel{m/min} \times \frac{0.1\ ml\ O_2/kg/min}{\cancel{m/min}} = 4.50\ ml\ O_2/kg/min$$

   Step 2: Find vert $\dot{V}O_2$.

$$\text{Vert } \dot{V}O_2 = .02 \times 45\ \cancel{m/min} \times \frac{1.8\ ml\ O_2/kg/min}{\cancel{m/min}} = 1.62\ ml\ O_2/kg/min$$

   Step 3: Rest $\dot{V}O_2 = 3.5\ ml\ O_2/kg/min$.

   Step 4: Add the three components together.

$$\begin{array}{rl} \text{Horiz } \dot{V}O_2 & = 4.50 \text{ ml } O_2/\text{kg/min} \\ \text{Vert } \dot{V}O_2 & = 1.62 \text{ ml } O_2/\text{kg/min} \\ + \text{ Rest } \dot{V}O_2 & = 3.50 \text{ ml } O_2/\text{kg/min} \\ \hline & 9.62 \text{ ml } O_2/\text{kg/min} = \text{total } \dot{V}O_2 \text{ (relative)} \\ & = 2.75 \text{ METs} \end{array}$$

Memory key: Only a relative $\dot{V}O_2$ can be converted directly to METs.

9. Speed = 80.4 m/min
   Horiz $\dot{V}O_2$ = 8.04 ml O_2/kg/min

   Vert $\dot{V}O_2$ = 5.7888 ml O_2/kg/min

   Total $\dot{V}O_2$ = 17.33 ml O_2/kg/min

10. Grade = 0.8 = 8%

    Math check: $\dfrac{9.8 \cancel{\text{ ml } O_2/\text{kg/min}}}{122.4 \cancel{\text{ ml } O_2/\text{kg/min}}} = .08$

11. Find percent grade. Math check: 53 × 1.8 = 95.4

    $\dfrac{19.2}{95.4} = .20 = 20\%$ grade

12. Find speed.

    Step 1: Subtract resting $\dot{V}O_2$.

    $$\begin{array}{rl} & 28.0 \text{ ml } O_2/\text{kg/min} \\ - & 3.5 \text{ ml } O_2/\text{kg/min} \\ \hline & 24.5 \text{ ml } O_2/\text{kg/min} = \text{horiz } \dot{V}O_2 + \text{vert } \dot{V}O_2 \end{array}$$

    Step 2: Add like terms. 0.1 + .162 = .262

    $$24.5 \text{ ml } O_2/\text{kg/min} = ?\text{ speed} \times 0.1 \; O_2/\text{kg/min} + ?\text{ speed} \times .09 \times 1.8 \text{ ml } O_2/\text{kg/min}$$

    Step 3: Isolate speed. Invert and perform the math.

    $$24.5 \text{ ml } O_2/\text{kg/min} = ?\text{ speed} \times \frac{.262 \text{ ml } O_2/\text{kg/min}}{\text{m/min}}$$

    $$24.5 \cancel{\text{ ml } O_2/\text{kg/min}} \times \frac{\text{m/min}}{.262 \cancel{\text{ ml } O_2/\text{kg/min}}} = 93.5 \text{ m/min}$$

13. Find speed. 84.56 m/min (approx 85 m/min)

    Math check: $\dfrac{11.5}{.136} = 84.56$

14. (a) 31.5 ml O_2/kg/min (relative)
    (b) 9 METs
    (c) 80 kg of body weight
    (d) 2,520 ml O_2/min (absolute)
    (e) 12.6 kcal/min
    (f) 693 kcal expended within 55 min

9 Oxygen Consumption During Running

Major Concepts

O_2 costs of running versus walking

Solving for total $\dot{V}O_2$

Solving for percent grade

Solving for speed

Evaluating treadmill belt speed

This chapter deals with the oxygen cost of running on a treadmill. Running differs from walking in that during running there is a period of flight (both feet off the ground) whereas during walking, one foot is always in contact with the ground. The ACSM metabolic equation for running described in this chapter can be used to estimate the energy cost of treadmill running and outdoor running on a level track under ideal weather conditions. The ACSM equation is not appropriate for hill running outdoors or for level running outdoors on rough or uneven surfaces or in the wind.

Comparing the O_2 Cost Equations for Running and Walking

Table 9.1 presents a comparison of the equations used to estimate the oxygen cost of running and walking. You will note that the equations differ only in the constants used for estimating the horizontal and vertical components. The constant for horizontal $\dot{V}O_2$ for running (.2 ml O_2/kg/min) is double the constant for walking (.1 ml O_2/kg/min). This reflects the fact that the toe push-off during running propels the runner along the horizontal plane, increasing the O_2 cost of the horizontal

Table 9.1 $\dot{V}O_2$ Components of the Walking and Running Equation

	Walking 50 to 100 m/min (1.87 to 3.73 mph)	**Running 80 to 134 m/min and faster (3.0 to 5.0 mph and faster)**
Horiz $\dot{V}O_2$	$\text{m/min} \times \frac{0.1 \text{ ml } O_2\text{/kg/min}}{\text{m/min}}$	$\text{m/min} \times \frac{0.2 \text{ ml } O_2\text{/kg/min}}{\text{m/min}}$
Vert $\dot{V}O_2$	$\text{\% grade} \times \text{m/min} \times \frac{1.8 \text{ ml } O_2\text{/kg/min}}{\text{m/min}}$	$\text{\% grade} \times \text{m/min} \times \frac{0.9 \text{ ml } O_2\text{/kg/min}}{\text{m/min}}$
Rest $\dot{V}O_2$	3.5 ml O_2/kg/min	3.5 ml O_2/kg/min

component while decreasing the O_2 cost of the vertical component. As shown, the vertical component for running (.9 ml O_2/kg/min divided by m/min) is about half that for walking (1.8 ml O_2/kg/min divided by m/min). As you might expect, the resting component of $\dot{V}O_2$ is the same for both equations.

Running and Walking Speeds

There is often confusion concerning whether the walking or running equation is more appropriate when the speed given is in that area (about 4 mph or 107.2 m/min) at which someone could be either walking or running. In these instances it would be necessary to observe the subject to determine whether walking or running mechanics were being used before one could select the correct equation. In the examples and practice problems for this chapter you will be told whether the subject is walking or running.

Calculating Energy Cost of Running

The calculations used for estimating the energy cost of running or for determining the percent grade and speed for a given energy cost are analogous to those used for walking. The examples that follow will illustrate these points.

Example 9A

Find total O_2 consumption and MET level. Jane is running on a treadmill at 4% grade and at a speed of 130 m/min. Determine her total O_2 consumption and METs.

Step 1: Determine horizontal $\dot{V}O_2$.

$$\text{Horiz } \dot{V}O_2 = 130 \cancel{\text{m/min}} \times \frac{0.2 \text{ ml } O_2\text{/kg/min}}{\cancel{\text{m/min}}}$$

$$\text{Horiz } \dot{V}O_2 = 26 \text{ ml } O_2\text{/kg/min}$$

Step 2: Determine vertical $\dot{V}O_2$.

$$\text{Vert } \dot{V}O_2 = .04 \times 130 \cancel{\text{m/min}} \times \frac{0.9 \text{ ml } O_2\text{/kg/min}}{\cancel{\text{m/min}}}$$

$$\text{Vert } \dot{V}O_2 = 4.68 \text{ ml } O_2\text{/kg/min}$$

Step 3: Add the three $\dot{V}O_2$ components.

$$\begin{aligned} \text{Horiz } \dot{V}O_2 &= \quad 26.0 \text{ ml } O_2/\text{kg/min} \\ \text{Vert } \dot{V}O_2 &= \quad 4.68 \text{ ml } O_2/\text{kg/min} \\ + \text{ Rest } \dot{V}O_2 &= + \ 3.50 \text{ ml } O_2/\text{kg/min} \\ \hline & \quad 34.18 \text{ ml } O_2/\text{kg/min} = \text{the total } \dot{V}O_2 \text{ for running} \end{aligned}$$

Step 4: Determine METs.

$$34.18 \ \cancel{\text{ml } O_2/\text{kg/min}} \times \frac{1 \text{ MET}}{3.5 \ \cancel{\text{ml } O_2/\text{kg/min}}} = 9.77 \text{ METs, almost 10}$$

Running at 4.85 mph (130 m/min) up a 4% grade yields a $\dot{V}O_2$ of about 34 ml O_2/kg/min at an intensity of about 10 METs.

Example 9B

Solve for percent grade. The exercise prescription for Mr. Hart suggests that he exercise at 46 ml O_2/kg/min (about 13 METs) for 10 min each day using a running (jogging) speed of 161 m/min. Determine the correct percent grade for the treadmill.

Step 1: Subtract the resting $\dot{V}O_2$ from the total $\dot{V}O_2$.

$$\begin{aligned} \text{Total } \dot{V}O_2 &= \quad 46.0 \text{ ml } O_2/\text{kg/min} \\ \text{Rest } \dot{V}O_2 &= - \ 3.5 \text{ ml } O_2/\text{kg/min} \\ \hline & \quad 42.5 \text{ ml } O_2/\text{kg/min} = \text{horiz } \dot{V}O_2 + \text{vert } \dot{V}O_2 \end{aligned}$$

Step 2: Calculate the horizontal component for running.

$$\text{Horiz } \dot{V}O_2 = 161 \ \cancel{\text{m/min}} \times \frac{0.2 \text{ ml } O_2/\text{kg/min}}{\cancel{\text{m/min}}}$$

$$\text{Horiz } \dot{V}O_2 = 32.2 \text{ ml } O_2/\text{kg/min}$$

Step 3: Subtract the horiz $\dot{V}O_2$ from the horiz + vert number to find the value of the vert $\dot{V}O_2$.

$$\begin{aligned} \text{Horiz } \dot{V}O_2 + \text{vert } \dot{V}O_2 &= \quad 42.5 \text{ ml } O_2/\text{kg/min} \\ \text{Horiz } \dot{V}O_2 &= - \ 32.2 \text{ ml } O_2/\text{kg/min} \\ \hline & \quad 10.3 \text{ ml } O_2/\text{kg/min} = \text{vert } \dot{V}O_2 \end{aligned}$$

Step 4: Fill in the equation. Use your pencil to cancel the units m/min.

(Vert $\dot{V}O_2$) (% grade) (Speed) (Constant)

$$10.3 \text{ ml } O_2/\text{kg/min} = \% \text{ grade} \times 161 \text{ m/min} \times \frac{0.9 \text{ ml } O_2/\text{kg/min}}{\text{m/min}}$$

$$10.3 \text{ ml } O_2/\text{kg/min} = \% \text{ grade} \times 144.9 \text{ ml } O_2/\text{kg/min}$$

Step 5: Divide both sides of the equation by 144.9 ml O_2/kg/min. Use your pencil to cancel the ml O_2/kg/min.

$$\frac{10.3 \text{ ml } O_2/\text{kg}/\text{min}}{144.9 \text{ ml } O_2/\text{kg}/\text{min}} = .071\text{, rounded to 7\% grade}$$

With a total $\dot{V}O_2$ of 46 ml O_2/kg/min (13 METs) and a running speed of 161 m/min (6 mph), the grade on the TM should be at 7% for Mr. Hart's 10-min run.

Example 9C

Solve for running speed. Jimmy has been prescribed exercise at about 13 to 14 METs (48 ml O_2/kg/min) for 8 min during the middle of his workout routine. When he is training at a 12% grade on the treadmill, what should his running speed be?

Step 1: Subtract the resting $\dot{V}O_2$ from the total $\dot{V}O_2$.

$$\begin{aligned} \text{Total } \dot{V}O_2 &= 48.0 \text{ ml } O_2/\text{kg}/\text{min} \\ \text{Rest } \dot{V}O_2 &= -3.5 \text{ ml } O_2/\text{kg}/\text{min} \\ \hline &44.5 \text{ ml } O_2/\text{kg}/\text{min} = \text{horiz } \dot{V}O_2 + \text{vert } \dot{V}O_2 \end{aligned}$$

Step 2: Rewrite the equation without the resting $\dot{V}O_2$.

$$44.5 \text{ ml } O_2/\text{kg}/\text{min} = ?\text{ speed} \times \frac{0.2 \text{ ml } O_2/\text{kg}/\text{min}}{\text{m}/\text{min}} + ?\text{ speed} \times .12 \times \frac{0.9 \text{ ml } O_2/\text{kg}/\text{min}}{\text{m}/\text{min}}$$

Step 3: Solve the equation.

(a) Multiply: $.12 \times 0.9 = .108$

(b) Add like terms $(0.2 + .108 = 0.308)$

(c) $(?\text{ speed} + ?\text{ speed} = ?\text{ speed})$

(d) $44.5 \text{ ml } O_2/\text{kg}/\text{min} = ?\text{ speed} \times \dfrac{0.308 \text{ ml } O_2/\text{kg}/\text{min}}{\text{m}/\text{min}}$

Step 4: Invert and multiply.

$$44.5 \cancel{\text{ml } O_2/\text{kg}/\text{min}} \times \frac{\text{m}/\text{min}}{0.308 \cancel{\text{ml } O_2/\text{kg}/\text{min}}} = 144.48 \text{ m}/\text{min} = \text{speed}$$

Step 5: Converting to mph.

$$144.48 \cancel{\text{m}/\text{min}} \times \frac{1 \text{ mph}}{26.8 \cancel{\text{m}/\text{min}}} = 5.39 \text{ mph, rounded to 5.4 mph}$$

With a total $\dot{V}O_2$ of 48 ml O_2/kg/min and a TM grade of 12%, the running speed would be 144.48 m/min, or 5.4 mph. The speed of 5.4 mph is a jog; this subject is using running-type mechanics, so the running equation is used.

Evaluating Treadmill Belt Speed Calibration

It is sometimes necessary to determine the accuracy of your treadmill speedometer, or to determine the speed of a treadmill that does not have a speedometer. To do this it is first necessary to determine the belt length of your treadmill (meters). This information is usually provided in the treadmill owner's manual. If not, unplug your treadmill and place a chalk mark on the belt and on the treadmill frame adjacent to the belt. Turn the belt one complete revolution while measuring the distance the chalk mark travels. Plug in the treadmill and turn it on at a desired speed. Determine the number of revolutions the belt makes per minute by counting the number of times the chalk mark on the belt passes the mark on the frame in 1 min (60 sec).

You can calculate the belt speed from:

$$\text{Speed (m/min)} = \text{belt length}\,\frac{\text{(m)}}{\text{rev}} \times \frac{\text{rev}}{\text{min}}$$

Convert speed in m/min to mph and compare to the treadmill set speed.

Example 9D

Determine the accuracy of a treadmill speedometer. Your treadmill is set at 7 mph. Is that speed accurate? You know the belt length is 5.55 m and you counted 34 belt rev/min at the 7-mph setting.

Step 1: Write the formula and solve.

$$\begin{aligned}\text{Speed m/min} &= \text{belt length}\,\frac{\text{(m)}}{\text{rev}} \times \frac{\text{rev}}{\text{min}}\\ &= \frac{5.55\ \text{m}}{\text{rev}} \times \frac{34\ \text{rev}}{\text{min}}\\ &= 188.7\ \text{m/min}\end{aligned}$$

Step 2: Convert m/min to mph.

$$188.7\ \text{m/min} \times \frac{1\ \text{mph}}{26.8\ \text{m/min}} = 7\ \text{mph}$$

The answer is *yes*, your treadmill is accurate at 7 mph. To perform a complete calibration check, you should complete this procedure at two or three other speeds. If the belt speed does not match the speedometer, consult your treadmill owner's manual for instructions on making adjustments to the speedometer needle.

Summary

Calculating total $\dot{V}O_2$ for running on a level treadmill involves adding the horizontal $\dot{V}O_2$ component to the resting $\dot{V}O_2$ component. To calculate total $\dot{V}O_2$ for running up a percent grade, the vertical $\dot{V}O_2$ component must be added to the equation. Checking the speed calibration of treadmills is a straightforward process and should be a routine procedure. The following practice problems will provide you with more understanding of the running $\dot{V}O_2$ mathematics and related calculations.

Chapter 9 Practice Problems

1. Convert the following to m/min.
   (a) 5 mph
   (b) 10 mph
2. What is 8 mph in terms of minutes/mile? And how long would it take to run 26.2 miles at this speed? (26.2 miles = a marathon)
3. Solve for the horizontal $\dot{V}O_2$ running component for each of the following.
   (a) 112 m/min
   (b) 8 mph
4. Solve for only the vertical $\dot{V}O_2$ running component for the following. Do not round off your answer at this point.
   (a) 2% grade, 186 m/min
   (b) 6% grade, 6.5 mph
5. Solve for total $\dot{V}O_2$ for running on a treadmill.
   Given 116 m/min and 5% grade, find total $\dot{V}O_2$ and METs.
6. Given the following information, which is the correct answer for total $\dot{V}O_2$? Running speed = 132 m/min and grade = 8%
   (a) 9.504 ml O_2/kg/min
   (b) 26.4 liters/kg/hr
   (c) 39.40 ml O_2/kg/min
   (d) 35.9 L/kg/min
7. Rocky is running on a level treadmill.
   Given horiz $\dot{V}O_2$ = 28 ml O_2/kg/min, find speed in m/min and mph.
8. Given total $\dot{V}O_2$ = 50 ml O_2/kg/min and grade = 4%, find speed in mph.
   Hint: When solving for speed on a graded treadmill you must always start with a total $\dot{V}O_2$.
9. Given total $\dot{V}O_2$ = 42 ml O_2/kg/min and grade = .02, find speed in m/min.
10. Given vert $\dot{V}O_2$ = 14.472 ml O_2/kg/min and speed = 268 m/min, find % grade.
11. Given total $\dot{V}O_2$ = 43.5 ml O_2/kg/min for running, find the value of (horiz $\dot{V}O_2$ + vert $\dot{V}O_2$).
12. Given total $\dot{V}O_2$ = 55.3 ml O_2/kg/min and speed = 228 m/min (8.5 mph), find % grade. (Review Example 9B).
13. Given total $\dot{V}O_2$ = 36 ml O_2/kg/min and speed = 115 m/min, find % grade.
14. Given total $\dot{V}O_2$ = 40 ml O_2/kg/min and grade = 6%, find speed. (Review Example 9C.)
15. Given total $\dot{V}O_2$ = 36 ml O_2/kg/min and grade = 8%, find speed.

16. During running on a treadmill at a 6% grade, Steve's total absolute $\dot{V}O_2$ is 2,520 ml O_2/min. Steve's weight is 70 kg. Find speed in m/min and mph.

17. Mr. Wright, who has a body weight of 176 lb, is running on the TM at a speed of 150 m/min at a 4% grade. Find relative $\dot{V}O_2$, absolute $\dot{V}O_2$, and METs.

18. A 25-year-old elite runner is running on a treadmill at 6 mph at a 20% grade. Determine $\dot{V}O_2$ and METs.

19. The runner in question 18 has a body weight of 70 kg. How many kcal is he expending per minute? First convert his relative $\dot{V}O_2$ to an absolute $\dot{V}O_2$.

    Use the conversion factor $\frac{.005 \text{ kcal}}{1 \text{ ml } O_2} = 1$ to determine kcal/min.

20. A treadmill has a belt that is 6.0 m in length. At the following belt revolutions per minute, determine belt speed in mph.

	Revolutions per minute	mph
(a)	22	?
(b)	28	?

21. Convert the following running speeds to mph.
    (a) 12 km/hr
    (b) 15 km/hr

22. Mr. Duncan, whose body weight is 70 kg, can run 2.42 kilometers in 12 min. Determine (a) through (g). Before performing any of the math, please read through the problem.
    (a) Running speed in mph
    (b) Running speed in m/min
    (c) Total $\dot{V}O_2$ (Use the level running equation.)
    (d) Approximate MET level of Mr. Duncan's run
    (e) Approximate absolute $\dot{V}O_2$
    (f) Approximate kcal expenditure per minute
    (g) Approximate kcal expenditure during the entire 12-min run

    No solution to this question will be given. Compare your answers with those of your colleagues.

    Hint: $\frac{1.5 \text{ miles}}{12 \text{ min}} \times \frac{60 \text{ min}}{1 \text{ hr}} = ?$

Chapter 9 Answers to Practice Problems

1. (a) $5 \cancel{\text{mph}} \times \frac{26.8 \text{ m/min}}{1 \cancel{\text{mph}}} = 134 \text{ m/min}$

   (b) 268.0 m/min

2. 8 mph $= \frac{8 \text{ miles}}{1 \text{ hr}}$, which inverted is $\frac{1 \text{ hr}}{8 \text{ miles}}$

   $\frac{1 \cancel{\text{hr}}}{8 \text{ miles}} \times \frac{60 \text{ min}}{1 \cancel{\text{hr}}} = \frac{7.5 \text{ min}}{\text{mile}}$ or 7 min and 30 sec

   Note: At 8 mph a runner would cover 1 mile in 7.5 min.

   $\frac{1 \text{ hr}}{8 \cancel{\text{miles}}} \times 26.2 \cancel{\text{miles}} = 3.275 \text{ hr} = 3 \text{ hr, } 16 \text{ min, } 30 \text{ sec}$

   $(.275 \cancel{\text{hr}} \times \frac{60 \text{ min}}{1 \cancel{\text{hr}}} = 16.5 \text{ min})$

3. Running. The horizontal $\dot{V}O_2$ components are as follows.
   (a) 22.4 ml O_2/kg/min
   (b) 42.88 ml O_2/kg/min

4. Running. The vertical $\dot{V}O_2$ components are as follows.
   (a) 3.348 ml O_2/kg/min
   (b) 9.4068 ml O_2/kg/min

5. Total $\dot{V}O_2$, running.

   $$\begin{aligned} \text{Horiz } \dot{V}O_2 &= \ 23.20 \text{ ml } O_2/\text{kg/min} \\ \text{Vert } \dot{V}O_2 &= \ \ 5.22 \text{ ml } O_2/\text{kg/min} \\ \text{Rest } \dot{V}O_2 &= +\ \ 3.5 \text{ ml } O_2/\text{kg/min} \\ \hline & \ 31.92 \text{ ml } O_2/\text{kg/min} = \text{total } \dot{V}O_2 = 9.12 \text{ METs} \end{aligned}$$

6. (c) 39.40 ml O_2/kg/min

7. Speed = 140 m/min, 5.22 mph

8. Find speed.

   Step 1: Find horiz + vert $\dot{V}O_2$.

   $$\begin{aligned} & 50.0 \text{ ml } O_2/\text{kg/min} \\ - & \ \ 3.5 \text{ ml } O_2/\text{kg/min} \\ \hline & 46.5 \text{ ml } O_2/\text{kg/min} = \text{horiz} + \text{vert } \dot{V}O_2 \end{aligned}$$

   Step 2: Set up the equation without the resting $\dot{V}O_2$.

   $$46.5 \text{ ml } O_2/\text{kg/min} = \text{speed} \times 0.2 \text{ ml } O_2/\text{kg/min} + \text{speed} \times .04 \times \frac{.9 \text{ ml } O_2/\text{kg/min}}{\text{m/min}}$$

   Step 3: Simplify the equation.

   $$46.5 \text{ ml } O_2/\text{kg/min} = \text{speed} \times \frac{.236 \text{ ml } O_2/\text{kg/min}}{\text{m/min}}$$

   $$46.5 \cancel{\text{ml } O_2/\text{kg/min}} \times \frac{\text{m/min}}{.236 \cancel{\text{ml } O_2/\text{kg/min}}} = 197 \text{ m/min}$$

9. 176.6 m/min

10. Grade: 0.06 = 6%

11. Total $\dot{V}O_2$ = 43.5 ml O_2/kg/min
    Rest $\dot{V}O_2$ = − 3.5 ml O_2/kg/min
    40.0 ml O_2/kg/min = horiz $\dot{V}O_2$ + vert $\dot{V}O_2$

12. Grade: 0.03 = 3%

13. Grade: 9% = 0.0917874

14. 143.7 m/min

    $$\text{Math check: } 36.5\ \cancel{\text{ml O}_2\text{/kg/min}} \times \frac{\text{m/min}}{.254\ \cancel{\text{ml O}_2\text{/kg/min}}} = 143.7\ \text{m/min}$$

15. 119.49 m/min

16. 127.95 m/min, or 4.77 mph

17. Relative $\dot{V}O_2$ = 38.90 ml O_2/kg/min = approximately 11.11 METs

    Absolute $\dot{V}O_2$ = 3,112 ml O_2/kg/min

18. 64.604 ml O_2/kg/min, or approximately 18.46 METs

19. $$\frac{64.604\ \text{ml O}_2}{\cancel{\text{kg}}\text{/min}} \times 70\ \cancel{\text{kg}} = 4{,}522.28\ \text{ml O}_2\text{/min}$$

    In order to convert to kcal/min we must use an absolute $\dot{V}O_2$.

    $$\frac{4522.28\ \cancel{\text{ml O}_2}}{\text{min}} \times \frac{.005\ \text{kcal}}{\cancel{\text{ml O}_2}} = \frac{22.6\ \text{kcal}}{\text{min}}$$

20. Converting TM belt revolutions/min to mph.

    (a) Step 1: Convert rev/min to m/min.

    $$\frac{22\ \cancel{\text{rev}}}{\text{min}} \times \frac{6\ \text{m}}{\cancel{\text{rev}}} = 132\ \text{m/min}$$

    Step 2: Convert m/min to mph.

    $$132\ \cancel{\text{m/min}} \times \frac{\text{mph}}{26.8\ \cancel{\text{m/min}}} = 4.93\ \text{mph}$$

    (b) 28 rev/min 6.27 mph

21. Finding mph

    (a) 7.44 mph

    (b) 9.3 mph

10 Cycle and Arm Ergometer Metabolic Equations

Major Concepts

Workload equations for the cycle and arm ergometer

Estimating total $\dot{V}O_2$ during cycle and arm exercise

Solving for workload in the units kgm/min

Solving for kg of cranking resistance

Finding the workload in kiloponds, Watts, kgm/min, and METs

Cycle and arm ergometers are widely used for physical work capacity testing as well as exercise training. To perform the math involving the cycle and arm ergometer equations, you need to consider units of resistance, workloads, and methods for estimating oxygen consumption.

The Mechanics of Leg and Arm Ergometers

There are two types of leg and arm ergometers—units that are mechanically braked and those that are electrically braked. Mechanically braked cycles and arm crank ergometers provide a constant resistance to the flywheel, but not a constant workload at varied pedaling speeds. As pedaling or arm cranking rate increases, workload increases, even with no change in the resistance.

In the electromagnetically braked unit, pedaling resistance is provided by increasing the field of current through the electromagnetic brake to the weighted flywheel. The pedaling rate can be varied without changing the overall pedaling resistance, because the electromagnet adjusts to varied pedaling rates to maintain a constant workload.

The mechanically braked ergometers, which are lighter and less expensive, are best suited for physical work capacity studies in field testing situations and less suited for daily exercise training. When these devices are used for daily exercise training the belts seem to wear considerably, changing the calibration of the ergometer and requiring replacement of the belt. In general, the electromagnetically braked leg and arm ergometers are better utilized as training equipment because they maintain calibration over long periods of usage.

The leg cycle ergometer has traditionally been viewed as an ideal piece of equipment for exercise testing. Because a cycle ergometer is stationary and because the subject remains seated, ECG electrodes and open-circuit spirometry for collection of expired gases can be attached to the subject more conveniently than when a subject is walking or running on a treadmill.

It is essential for the exercise professional to be able to calculate ergometer workloads and estimate oxygen consumption values based upon cranking resistance and speed of cranking. Many fitness facilities perform submaximal and maximal aerobic capacity assessments using the cycle ergometer; and for subjects who are unable to use their legs or who are involved in an occupation that requires a great deal of arm activity, an arm ergometer can be used for testing or for daily training. You will read about exercise testing in chapter 12.

Workload Calculations for the Leg and Arm Ergometer

The workload for leg and arm ergometers is expressed in kgm/min. To calculate kgm/min, use this equation, based upon *cranking resistance of the pedals*, the *distance the flywheel travels* in one revolution of the pedals, and the *number of revolutions per minute* of the pedals or arm crank handles.

$$\frac{\text{kgm}}{\text{min}} = \frac{\text{kg}}{1} \times \frac{\text{m}}{\text{rev}} \times \frac{\text{rev}}{\text{min}}$$

where,

(a) kgm/min is the basic workload unit for leg and arm ergometry (1 kgm/min requires approximately 1.8 ml O_2/min);
(b) kg (kilogram) is the amount of resistance applied to the flywheel (the kp, or kilopond, is used interchangeably with kg; we will use both in this text);
(c) m/rev is the distance the flywheel travels per pedal revolution (the m/rev is 6 for the Monark and 3 for the Tunturi and Bodyguard ergometers);
(d) rev/min (rpm) is the speed at which the pedals are turned (most cycle or arm test protocols use 50 rev/min; for training, pedaling speed can vary from 30 to 110 rev/min).

Note also that workload is sometimes expressed in Watts. The conversion factor is

$$\frac{6\ \text{kgm/min}}{1\ \text{Watt}} \text{ or } \frac{1\ \text{Watt}}{6\ \text{kgm/min}}$$

Table 10.1 gives equivalents between Watts and kgm/min.

The equation for determining ergometer workload (kg) can be rearranged to calculate cranking resistance. Notice how m/rev and rev/min are inverted in this equation:

$$\frac{\text{kg}}{1} = \frac{\text{kgm}}{\text{min}} \times \frac{\text{rev}}{\text{m}} \times \frac{\text{min}}{\text{rev}}$$

The example problems here will provide you with the concepts needed for calculating workloads for leg and arm exercise. You will use the kgm/min values in the leg and arm equations when calculating total $\dot{V}O_2$. As you work through the problems in this chapter, make a point of locating the appropriate information on Tables 10.1 and 10.2 on pages 120 and 125. You will find these tables useful for finding workloads and METs.

Example 10A

Solve for leg or arm workloads. You are pedaling with 2 kg of pedal resistance on a cycle ergometer that has a flywheel distance of 6 m/rev. You are pedaling at 60 rev/min. Find kgm/min and Watts.

Step 1: Write the equation and enter the known values.

$$\text{kgm/min} = \frac{\text{kg}}{1} \times \frac{\text{m}}{\text{rev}} \times \frac{\text{rev}}{\text{min}}$$

$$= \frac{2\ \text{kg}}{1} \times \frac{6\ \text{m}}{\cancel{\text{rev}}} \times \frac{60\ \cancel{\text{rev}}}{\text{min}}$$

$$= 720\ \text{kgm/min}$$

Step 2: Convert the workload answer into Watts.

$$720\ \cancel{\text{kgm/min}} \times \frac{1\ \text{Watt}}{6\ \cancel{\text{kgm/min}}} = 120\ \text{Watts}$$

Compare the above with the values in Table 10.1. Find 60 rpm and 2 kg.

Example 10B

Calculate kilograms of cranking/pedaling resistance. Jason is cranking an arm ergometer at 450 kgm/min (75 Watts). The flywheel travels 6 m in one revolution of a pedal. His cranking speed is 50 rev/min. Find the pedal resistance in both kg and lb.

Step 1: Write the formula and enter the known values.

$$\text{kg of resistance} = \frac{\text{kgm}}{\text{min}} \times \frac{\text{rev}}{\text{m}} \times \frac{\text{min}}{\text{rev}}$$

Step 2: Enter the given values into the equation. Cancel the appropriate units; then multiply.

$$\text{kg} = \frac{450\ \text{kg}\cancel{\text{m}}}{\cancel{\text{min}}} \times \frac{1\ \cancel{\text{rev}}}{6\ \cancel{\text{m}}} \times \frac{1\ \cancel{\text{min}}}{50\ \cancel{\text{rev}}}$$

$$\text{kg} = 1.50\ \text{kg of pedal resistance}$$

Compare this 1.50 kg of resistance and 50 rpm with values in Table 10.1. Can you find where the 450 kgm/min is located between 300 and 600?

Step 3: Convert kg to lb.

$$1.50\ \cancel{\text{kg}} \times \frac{2.2\ \text{lb}}{1\ \cancel{\text{kg}}} = 3.3\ \text{lb of pedaling resistance}$$

Table 10.1 Table of Watts and kgm/min Based Upon Arm and Leg rev/min and kg of Pedaling Resistance

		kg (kp)							
rev/min		**0.25**	**0.5**	**1**	**2**	**3**	**4**	**5**	**6**
30	Watts	7.5	15	30	60	90	120	150	180
	kgm/min	45	90	180	360	540	720	900	1,080
40	Watts	10	20	40	80	120	160	200	240
	kgm/min	60	120	240	480	720	960	1,200	1,440
50	Watts	12.5	25	50	100	150	200	250	300
	kgm/min	75	150	300	600	900	1,200	1,500	1,800
60	Watts	15	30	60	120	180	240	300	360
	kgm/min	90	180	360	720	1,080	1,440	1,800	2,160
70	Watts	17.5	35	70	140	210	280	350	420
	kgm/min	105	210	420	840	1,260	1,680	2,100	2,520
80	Watts	20	40	80	160	240	320	400	480
	kgm/min	120	240	480	960	1,440	1,920	2,400	2,880
90	Watts	22.5	45	90	180	270	360	450	540
	kgm/min	135	270	540	1,080	1,620	2,160	2,700	3,240
100	Watts	25	50	100	200	300	400	500	600
	kgm/min	150	300	600	1,200	1,800	2,400	3,000	3,600
110	Watts	27.5	55	110	220	330	440	550	660
	kgm/min	165	330	660	1,320	1,980	2,640	3,300	3,960

Estimating Total $\dot{V}O_2$ During Cycle and Arm Exercise

We will begin by looking at the ACSM equations for estimating total $\dot{V}O_2$ during cycle and arm exercises.

ACSM Cycle Equation

$$\text{Total } \dot{V}O_2 = \left(\frac{\text{kgm}}{\text{min}} \times \frac{2 \text{ ml } O_2}{\text{kgm}}\right) + \left(\frac{3.5 \text{ ml } O_2}{\text{kg/min}} \times \frac{\text{body wt (kg)}}{1}\right)$$

This equation is most accurate at workloads from 300 kgm/min (50 Watts) to 1,200 kgm/min (200 Watts). Calculations using workloads up to 4,200 kgm/min can be performed but with decreased accuracy.

ACSM Arm Ergometer Equation

$$\text{Total } \dot{V}O_2 = \left(\frac{\text{kgm}}{\text{min}} \times \frac{3 \text{ ml } O_2}{\text{kgm}}\right) + \left(\frac{3.5 \text{ ml } O_2}{\text{kg/min}} \times \frac{\text{body wt (kg)}}{1}\right)$$

This equation is most accurate between 150 kgm/min (23 Watts) and 750 kgm/min (125 Watts).

The only difference between the arm and leg equations is that the resistance $\dot{V}O_2$ for arm ergometry (3 ml O_2/kgm) is slightly higher than for leg cycling (2 ml O_2/kgm) due to the additional musculature of the shoulders, back, and chest needed to stabilize the upper extremities while cranking (ACSM, 1995).

A number of investigators have gathered evidence to explain the difference in O_2 requirements between arm and leg exercise. Arm cranking exercise produces a greater cardiovascular strain, an increasing peripheral resistance, and a slightly slower venous blood return due to a greater isometric component over that seen in leg cranking exercise (Astrand & Rodahl, 1986; Bevegard, 1966; Bevegard & Shepard, 1967; Fardy, 1977; Franklin, 1982b; Franklin, 1983). For a comprehensive discussion comparing the physiological responses of arm versus leg cranking exercise, see also Toner, Glickman, & McArdle (1990).

Recent studies (Latin, Berg, Smith, Tolle, & Woodby-Brown, 1993; Berry, Storsteen, & Woodard, 1993) are suggesting cycle equations slightly different from the ACSM equations (ACSM, 1995). These two equations are as follows.

The Latin Equation

$$\dot{V}O_2 \text{ (ml } O_2\text{/min)} = (\text{kgm/min} \times 1.98 \text{ ml } O_2\text{/min}) + \left((3.5 \text{ ml } O_2\text{/kg/min} \times \text{kg body wt}) + (260 \text{ ml } O_2\text{/min})\right)$$

The Berry Equation

$$\dot{V}O_2 \text{ (ml } O_2\text{/min)} = (10.9 \times \text{Watts}) + (8.2 \times \text{pedaling rev/min}) + (8.3 \times \text{kg body wt}) - (559.60)$$

Both of these equations use the same basic concepts and principles as the ACSM equations. After completing this chapter and practice problems you should be able to perform the Latin and Berry equations with little difficulty.

Further studies are needed to resolve the slight discrepancy between the ACSM cycle equations and the Latin and Berry equations. Until the ACSM officially publishes either of the equations by Latin or Berry in the *Guidelines For Exercise Testing and Prescription* (ACSM, 1995) for certification or college exams, you should continue to use the ACSM equations.

You may wonder why body weight is used in the cycle and arm equations and not in the bench stepping or treadmill equations. On a treadmill, total relative $\dot{V}O_2$ (ml O_2/kg/min) can be estimated on the basis of speed and percent grade. Body weight is not considered because the individual is carrying his or her own body weight while walking or running and contributes to the amount of work being performed. Body weight in kilograms is already included as part of the total $\dot{V}O_2$.

On a cycle or arm ergometer, in contrast, absolute $\dot{V}O_2$ (ml O_2/min) is estimated on the basis of a subject's weight, pedaling resistance, and pedaling speed. While they are cycling or arm cranking, people are not supporting their own body weight. Body weight is supported by the seat and handle bars. Thus, the body weight has no influence upon the cycle workload.

Cycle Ergometry Example Problems

The ACSM cycle and arm ergometer equations can be used to estimate total $\dot{V}O_2$ when workload is known or to estimate workload when total $\dot{V}O_2$ is known. The examples and the practice problems for this chapter will help you better understand these calculations.

The cycle ergometer is used in most fitness and rehabilitation facilities for both exercise training and exercise testing. The metabolic equation for estimating oxygen consumption during cycling is very useful in both of these contexts. The leg cycle equation, like the arm cycle equation, can be used to estimate total $\dot{V}O_2$ when the workload is known or to estimate workload when total $\dot{V}O_2$ is known. The following examples illustrate these calculations.

Example 10C

Find oxygen consumption, kcal/min, and METs for a cycle ergometer. John weighs 80 kg and is riding a Monark cycle ergometer at 50 rev/min at a workload of 200 Watts (1,200 kgm/min). Estimate his absolute $\dot{V}O_2$, kcal/min, relative $\dot{V}O_2$, and MET level.

Step 1: Write out the formula and substitute known values.

$$\text{Total } \dot{V}O_2 = \left(\text{workload } \frac{\text{kgm}}{\text{min}} \times \frac{2 \text{ ml } O_2}{\text{kgm}}\right) + \left(\frac{3.5 \text{ ml } O_2}{\text{kg/min}} \times \text{kg}\right)$$

$$= \left(\frac{1{,}200 \cancel{\text{kgm}}}{\text{min}} \times \frac{2 \text{ ml } O_2}{\cancel{\text{kgm}}}\right) + \left(\frac{3.5 \text{ ml } O_2}{\cancel{\text{kg}}/\text{min}} \times 80 \cancel{\text{kg}}\right)$$

Step 2: Perform calculation.

$$\text{Total } \dot{V}O_2 = \frac{2{,}400 \text{ ml } O_2}{\text{min}} + \frac{280 \text{ ml } O_2}{\text{min}}$$

$$\text{Total } \dot{V}O_2 = \frac{2{,}680 \text{ ml } O_2}{\text{min}} \quad (\text{absolute } \dot{V}O_2)$$

Step 3: Use the conversion factor .005 kcal/ml O_2 to solve for kcal/min. The units ml O_2 cancel.

$$\frac{2{,}680 \cancel{\text{ml } O_2}}{\text{min}} \times \frac{.005 \text{ kcal}}{\cancel{\text{ml } O_2}} = 13.4 \text{ kcal/min}$$

Step 4: Convert absolute to relative $\dot{V}O_2$ by dividing absolute $\dot{V}O_2$ by body weight (kg).

$$\frac{2{,}680 \text{ ml } O_2/\text{min}}{80 \text{ kg}} = 33.5 \text{ ml } O_2/\text{kg/min}$$

Step 5: Convert to METs.

$$33.5 \cancel{\text{ml } O_2/\text{kg/min}} \times \frac{1 \text{ MET}}{3.5 \cancel{\text{ml } O_2/\text{kg/min}}} = 9.57 \text{ METs}$$

Example 10D

Solve for $\dot{V}O_2$ based upon kg (kp) of pedaling resistance, distance the flywheel travels with one pedal revolution, and pedaling rev/min. Ms. Jansen, a 56-kg woman, performed a maximal effort on a Monark cycle ergometer at a resistance of 3 kg and a pedal rate of 60 rev/min. What were her absolute $\dot{V}O_2$, relative $\dot{V}O_2$, and MET level? (Remember that the Monark ergometer flywheel travels 6 m/rev.)

Step 1: Calculate workload by substituting known values into the workload equation.

$$\text{workload}\ \frac{\text{kgm}}{\text{min}} = \frac{\text{resistance (kg)}}{1} \times \frac{\text{m}}{\text{rev}} \times \frac{\text{rev}}{\text{min}}$$

$$= \frac{3\ \text{kg}}{1} \times \frac{6\ \text{m}}{\cancel{\text{rev}}} \times \frac{60\ \cancel{\text{rev}}}{\text{min}}$$

$$\text{workload}\ \frac{\text{kgm}}{\text{min}} = 1{,}080\ \text{kgm/min}$$

Step 2: Calculate total absolute $\dot{V}O_2$ by substituting known values into the cycle equation.

$$\dot{V}O_2 = \left(\text{workload}\ \frac{\text{kgm}}{\text{min}} \times \frac{2\ \text{ml O}_2}{\text{kgm}}\right) + \left(\frac{3.5\ \text{ml O}_2}{\cancel{\text{kg}}/\text{min}} \times \cancel{\text{kg}}\right)$$

$$= \left(\frac{1{,}080\ \text{kgm}}{\text{min}} \times \frac{2\ \text{ml O}_2}{\text{kgm}}\right) + \left(\frac{3.5\ \text{ml O}_2}{\cancel{\text{kg}}/\text{min}} \times 56\ \cancel{\text{kg}}\right)$$

$$= 2{,}160\ \frac{\text{ml O}_2}{\text{min}} + 196\ \frac{\text{ml O}_2}{\text{min}}$$

$$= 2{,}356\ \frac{\text{ml O}_2}{\text{min}}\ \text{(absolute)}$$

Step 3: Calculate relative $\dot{V}O_2$ by dividing absolute $\dot{V}O_2$ by body weight.

$$\frac{2{,}356\ \text{ml O}_2/\text{min}}{56\ \text{kg}} = 42.07\ \text{ml O}_2/\text{kg/min}$$

Step 4: Convert to METs.

$$42.07\ \cancel{\text{ml O}_2/\text{kg/min}} \times \frac{1\ \text{MET}}{3.5\ \cancel{\text{ml O}_2/\text{kg/min}}} = 12.02\ \text{METs}$$

When solving for total $\dot{V}O_2$, as in Example 10D, the resting $\dot{V}O_2$ is added to the resistive $\dot{V}O_2$. When solving for workload, the resting $\dot{V}O_2$ must first be subtracted from the total $\dot{V}O_2$, as in the next example.

Example 10E

Calculate the workload for a given oxygen consumption. The maximal measured O_2 uptake for Mr. Sexton, a 68-kg man, was 3,500 ml O_2/min. His exercise prescription calls for cycle ergometer training at 80% of his $\dot{V}O_2$max. What is the prescribed workload in kgm/min and Watts?

Step 1: Calculate training $\dot{V}O_2$ at 80% of max.

$$.80 \times 3{,}500\ \text{ml O}_2/\text{min} = 2{,}800\ \text{ml O}_2/\text{min}$$

Step 2: Write out the leg cycle $\dot{V}O_2$ equation and substitute known values.

Total $\dot{V}O_2$ (Resistive component) (Resting component)

$$\frac{2{,}800 \text{ ml } O_2}{\text{min}} = \left(\frac{?\text{ kgm}}{\text{min}} \times \frac{2 \text{ ml } O_2}{\text{kgm}}\right) + \left(\frac{3.5 \text{ ml } O_2}{\text{kg/min}} \times \frac{68 \text{ kg}}{1}\right)$$

Step 3: To solve for workload we must subtract the rest $\dot{V}O_2$ from the total $\dot{V}O_2$. First the rest $\dot{V}O_2$ must be converted to an absolute $\dot{V}O_2$.

(Relative rest $\dot{V}O_2$) (Absolute rest $\dot{V}O_2$)

$$\frac{3.5 \text{ ml } O_2}{\cancel{\text{kg}}/\text{min}} \times \frac{68 \cancel{\text{kg}}}{1} = \frac{238 \text{ ml } O_2}{\text{min}}$$

Step 4: Subtract the rest $\dot{V}O_2$ from the total $\dot{V}O_2$.

$$\begin{aligned} \text{Total } \dot{V}O_2 &= \quad 2{,}800 \text{ ml } O_2/\text{min} \\ \text{Rest } \dot{V}O_2 &= - \quad 238 \text{ ml } O_2/\text{min} \\ & \quad\ \ 2{,}562 \text{ ml } O_2/\text{min} = \text{resistive } \dot{V}O_2 \end{aligned}$$

Step 5: Write out the resistive component.

(Resistive $\dot{V}O_2$ component)

$$\frac{2{,}562 \text{ ml } O_2}{\text{min}} = \frac{?\text{ kgm}}{\text{min}} \times \frac{2 \text{ ml } O_2}{\text{kgm}}$$

Step 6: Invert the 2 ml O_2/kgm and multiply. The ml O_2 cancel.

$$\frac{2{,}562 \cancel{\text{ml } O_2}}{\text{min}} \times \frac{\text{kgm}}{2 \cancel{\text{ml } O_2}} = \frac{1{,}281 \text{ kgm}}{\text{min}}$$

Step 7: Convert to Watts. The kgm/min cancel.

$$1{,}281 \cancel{\text{kgm/min}} \times \frac{1 \text{ Watt}}{6 \cancel{\text{kgm/min}}} = 213.5 \text{ Watts}$$

On a Monark cycle the resistance would be set at about 200 Watts with a pedaling speed of 50 rev/min. On an Air-Dyne cycle the subject would ride at a speedometer setting of just a little faster than #4 on the dial, which represents 4 kg (4 kp) of pedaling resistance.

Table 10.2 provides a quick reference for obtaining MET levels based upon body weight and workloads on a cycle ergometer. You can compare your practice problem answers with the MET levels listed. This table will help you when prescribing workloads for subjects who pedal or arm crank at a variety of rev/min.

Table 10.2 MET Table for Cycle Ergometers

		.5 150 25	1 300 50	 450 75	2 600 100	 750 125	3 900 150	 1,050 175	4 1,200 200	 1,350 225	5 1,500 250	 1,650 275	6 1,800 300	kp (kg) kgm/min Watts
kg	lbs													
40	88	3.2	5.3	7.4	9.6	11.7	13.9	16.1	18.9	21.6	24.0	26.6	29.2	
45	99	2.9	4.8	6.7	8.6	10.5	12.4	14.4	16.9	19.3	21.6	23.7	26.0	
50	110	2.8	4.4	6.1	7.8	9.5	11.2	12.9	15.3	17.5	19.5	21.5	23.5	
55	121	2.6	4.1	5.7	7.3	8.8	10.4	11.9	14.0	16.0	17.8	19.6	21.5	
60	132	2.5	3.8	5.3	6.7	8.2	9.6	11.0	12.9	14.8	16.4	18.1	19.8	
65	143	2.4	3.6	4.9	6.3	7.6	8.9	10.2	12.0	13.7	15.2	16.7	18.3	
70	154	2.3	3.4	4.6	5.9	7.1	8.3	9.6	11.2	12.8	14.2	15.6	17.1	
75	165	2.2	3.3	4.4	5.6	6.7	7.9	9.0	10.6	12.0	13.3	14.6	16.0	
80	176	2.1	3.1	4.2	5.3	6.4	7.4	8.5	9.9	11.3	12.6	13.8	15.1	
85	187	2.0	3.0	4.0	5.0	6.0	7.1	8.1	9.4	10.7	11.9	13.0	14.3	
90	198	1.9	2.9	3.8	4.8	5.8	6.7	7.7	9.0	10.2	11.3	12.4	13.5	
95	209	1.8	2.8	3.7	4.6	5.5	6.4	7.4	8.5	9.7	10.7	11.8	12.9	
100	220	1.8	2.7	3.6	4.4	5.3	6.2	7.0	8.1	9.3	10.3	11.2	12.3	
105	231	1.8	2.6	3.4	4.3	5.1	5.9	6.7	7.8	8.9	9.8	10.7	11.7	
110	242	1.7	2.5	3.3	4.1	4.9	5.7	6.5	7.5	8.5	9.4	10.3	11.2	
115	253	1.7	2.4	3.2	4.0	4.7	5.5	6.2	7.2	8.2	9.0	10.0	10.8	
120	264	1.7	2.4	3.1	3.9	4.6	5.3	6.0	7.0	7.9	8.7	9.5	10.4	
125	276	1.6	2.3	3.0	3.8	4.4	5.1	5.8	6.7	7.6	8.4	9.2	10.0	
130	286	1.6	2.3	2.9	3.6	4.3	4.9	5.6	6.5	7.3	8.1	8.9	9.7	
135	297	1.6	2.2	2.8	3.5	4.2	4.8	5.4	6.3	7.1	7.9	8.6	9.3	
140	309	1.6	2.2	2.7	3.4	4.1	4.6	5.3	6.1	6.9	7.6	8.3	9.0	

Arm Ergometry Example Problems

The next series of example problems will concentrate on the arm ergometer metabolic equation. In examples 10F and 10G we will solve for total $\dot{V}O_2$. Example 10H shows how to find the workload (kgm/min) when you are provided with the total $\dot{V}O_2$ value. As you examine these examples, use your pencil to cancel out the appropriate units.

Example 10F

Find total $\dot{V}O_2$ for arm ergometer; find kcal/min and METs. Mr. Jones, who weighs 95 kg, is using an arm crank ergometer at a workload of 450 kgm/min at 50 rev/min. What is the total oxygen consumption? What is the energy expenditure in kcal/min and in METs?

Step 1: Write out the equation and substitute known values.

$$\text{Total } \dot{V}O_2 = \text{workload } \frac{(\text{kgm})}{\text{min}} \times \frac{3 \text{ ml } O_2}{\text{kgm}} + \frac{3.5 \text{ ml } O_2}{\text{kg/min}} \times \frac{\text{body wt (kg)}}{1}$$

$$= \frac{450 \text{ kgm}}{\text{min}} \times \frac{3 \text{ ml } O_2}{\text{kgm}} + \frac{3.5 \text{ ml } O_2}{\text{kg/min}} \times 95 \text{ kg}$$

Step 2: Solve.

$$= \frac{1{,}350 \text{ ml } O_2}{\text{min}} + \frac{332.5 \text{ ml } O_2}{\text{min}}$$

$$\text{Total } \dot{V}O_2 = \frac{1{,}682.5 \text{ ml } O_2}{\text{min}}$$

(an absolute VO_2, i.e., not relative to body weight)

Step 3: Convert the absolute VO_2 to kcal/min of energy expenditure. Use .005 kcal/ml O_2 as the conversion factor.

$$\frac{1{,}682.5 \cancel{\text{ ml } O_2}}{\text{min}} \times \frac{.005 \text{ kcal}}{\cancel{\text{ml } O_2}} = \frac{8.41 \text{ kcal}}{\text{min}} \text{ (about 8.4 kcal/min)}$$

Step 4: Convert the absolute $\dot{V}O_2$ to a relative VO_2. Divide the absolute $\dot{V}O_2$ by Mr. Jones' body weight.

$$\frac{1{,}682.5 \text{ ml } O_2/\text{min}}{95 \text{ kg}} = 17.71 \text{ ml } O_2/\text{kg/min}$$

Step 5: Convert the relative $\dot{V}O_2$ of 17.7 ml O_2/kg/min to METs.

$$17.7 \cancel{\text{ ml } O_2/\text{kg/min}} \times \frac{1 \text{ MET}}{3.5 \cancel{\text{ ml } O_2/\text{kg/min}}} = 5.06 \text{ METs}$$

At an arm cranking workload resistance of 450 kgm/min with a subject weighing 95 kg, the absolute $\dot{V}O_2$ is 1,682.5 ml O_2/min, the relative $\dot{V}O_2$ is 17.71 ml O_2/kg/min, and the energy expenditure is about 8.4 kcal/min at 5.06 METs. Note that the only way to convert from kgm/min to total $\dot{V}O_2$ and METs is by using the arm or the leg ergometer equation.

Example 10G

Prescribe a workload. Mike (a 68-kg man who exercises in his wheelchair) has just completed a GXT on an arm ergometer at 50 rev/min. His exercise prescription calls for arm cranking at a $\dot{V}O_2$ of 2,215 ml O_2/min. What is the appropriate workload in Watts?

Step 1: Set up the equation.

$$(\text{Total } \dot{V}O_2) = (\text{resistive } \dot{V}O_2) + (\text{rest } \dot{V}O_2)$$

$$2{,}215 \text{ ml } O_2/\text{min} = \left(\frac{? \text{ kgm}}{\text{min}} \times \frac{3 \text{ ml } O_2}{\text{kgm}}\right) + \left(\frac{3.5 \text{ ml } O_2}{\text{kg/min}} \times \frac{68 \text{ kg}}{1}\right)$$

Step 2: Convert the resting $\dot{V}O_2$ to an absolute $\dot{V}O_2$.

$$\frac{3.5 \text{ ml } O_2}{\cancel{\text{kg}}/\text{min}} \times \frac{68 \cancel{\text{kg}}}{1} = \frac{238 \text{ ml } O_2}{\text{min}}$$

Step 3: Subtract the resting $\dot{V}O_2$ from the total $\dot{V}O_2$.

$$\begin{aligned} \text{Total } \dot{V}O_2 &= \quad 2{,}215 \text{ ml } O_2/\text{min} \\ \text{Rest } \dot{V}O_2 &= -\ \ 238 \text{ ml } O_2/\text{min} \\ \hline & \quad 1{,}977 \text{ ml } O_2/\text{min} = \text{resistive } \dot{V}O_2 \end{aligned}$$

Step 4: The resistive $\dot{V}O_2$ component now looks like this.

$$1{,}977 \text{ ml } O_2/\text{min} = \frac{? \text{ kgm}}{\text{min}} \times \frac{3 \text{ ml } O_2}{\text{kgm}}$$

Invert the 3 ml O_2/kgm and multiply times the 1,977 ml O_2/min. The ml O_2 cancel.

$$\frac{1{,}977 \cancel{\text{ml } O_2}}{\text{min}} \times \frac{\text{kgm}}{3 \cancel{\text{ml } O_2}} = \frac{659 \text{ kgm}}{\text{min}}$$

Step 5: Convert the workload of 659 kgm/min into Watts.

$$659 \cancel{\text{kgm/min}} \times \frac{1 \text{ Watt}}{6 \cancel{\text{kgm/min}}} = 109.83 \text{ Watts (about 110 W)}$$

For training, Mike should be turning the arm crank using a workload of about 110 Watts, which is a resistance of slightly more than 2 kg (or 2 kp). According to Table 10.1, Mike can vary his arm cranking speed and still maintain the workload of about 110 Watts. At 50 rev/min, 2 kp is 100 Watts; 100 Watts can also be achieved at a setting of 1 kp with a cranking speed of 100 rev/min.

Example 10H

Solve for total $\dot{V}O_2$ when kgm/min is unknown. We will first solve for kgm/min. Then, using the arm equation, we will solve for total $\dot{V}O_2$.

Given 2 kg of pedal resistance (100 Watts), 6 m/rev of flywheel distance, 60 rev/min of pedaling speed, and an 80-kg subject, find kgm/min, Watts, and total $\dot{V}O_2$.

Step 1: Enter values into the workload equation, cancel, and multiply.

$$? \frac{\text{kg}}{1} \times \frac{?\ \text{m}}{\text{rev}} \times \frac{?\ \text{rev}}{\text{min}} = ?\ \text{kgm/min}$$

$$\frac{2\ \text{kg}}{1} \times \frac{6\ \text{m}}{\cancel{\text{rev}}} \times \frac{60\ \cancel{\text{rev}}}{\text{min}} = \frac{720\ \text{kgm}}{\text{min}}$$

Step 2: Convert kgm/min to Watts.

$$720\ \cancel{\text{kgm/min}} \times \frac{1\ \text{Watt}}{6\ \cancel{\text{kgm/min}}} = 120\ \text{Watts}$$

Step 3: Insert the workload 720 kgm/min into the arm ergometer equation and then solve for total $\dot{V}O_2$. Use your pencil to cancel the appropriate units; then add.

$$\text{Resistive } \dot{V}O_2 = \frac{720\ \text{kgm}}{\text{min}} \times \frac{3\ \text{ml } O_2}{\text{kgm}} = 2{,}160\ \text{ml } O_2/\text{min}$$

$$\text{Rest } \dot{V}O_2 = \frac{3.5\ \text{ml } O_2}{\text{kg/min}} \times \frac{80\ \text{kg}}{1} = +\ 280\ \text{ml } O_2/\text{min}$$

$$\text{Total } \dot{V}O_2 = 2{,}440\ \text{ml } O_2/\text{min}$$

Ergometer Workloads Relative to Pedaling Speed

Stationary cycle ergometers such as the Schwinn Air-Dyne and the Monark cycles display the workloads in units of Watts, kgm/min, and kp (or kg) on a dial or gauge. On a mechanically braked cycle like the Monark, when the resistance is set on a specific workload, 2 kp for example, the workload of 600 kgm/min is correct only when the subject is pedaling at the standard 50 rpm. When a subject pedals faster than 50 rpm, the workload (work of pedaling) increases, even though the dial still reads 2 kp. Every exercise professional should have a complete understanding of this important concept when designing exercise prescriptions.

Table 10.1 illustrates the effect of varied rev/min (rpm) of pedaling speed upon kgm/min. When the workload on a mechanically braked cycle is set at 1 kp and the pedaling speed is 50 rev/min, the workload is 300 kgm/min, as you can see in Table 10.1. When the workload is set at 1 kp but the pedaling speed is changed to 80 rev/min, the workload actually becomes 480 kgm/min.

Use Tables 10.1 and 10.2 to follow this example:

A subject is pedaling at 100 rev/min with a pedaling resistance of 2 kp. Table 10.1 shows that this is a workload of 1,200 kgm/min. Table 10.2 shows that 1200 kgm/min for a 95-kg subject is an exercise intensity of 8.5 METs.

A second subject is pedaling at 50 rev/min at 4 kp, yielding a workload of 1,200 kgm/min (200 Watts, Table 10.1). From Table 10.2 we see that this cycle setting (1200 kgm/min) for a 75-kg subject would convert to an intensity level of approximately 10.6 METs.

Summary

An important aspect of exercise physiology is the measurement and prescription of workloads. The cycle and the arm crank ergometer allow workloads to be measured very accurately. With these ergometers, body weight is not a variable.

Chapter 10 Practice Problems

1. Convert the following body weights to kg.

   (a) 140 lb

   (b) 185 lb

2. Convert the following body weights in kg to lb.

   (a) 92 kg

   (b) 65 kg

Practice problems 3 through 15 pertain to the cycle ergometer.

3. An 84-kg man is riding a Tunturi cycle at a workload of 1,500 kgm/min. Find the absolute $\dot{V}O_2$ and the MET level.

4. A 176-lb man is riding a Monark cycle at a workload of 225 Watts. Find the absolute $\dot{V}O_2$. Also, how many kcal/min is he expending at this workload?

5. John, a 105-kg man, is riding a Bodyguard cycle and consuming a total $\dot{V}O_2$ of 1,890 ml O2/min. Find METs.

6. John (105 kg) is now riding a cycle at 125 Watts. Find METs.

7. Convert the absolute $\dot{V}O_2$ of 1,869 ml O2/min into kcal/min.

8. Mary, a professional wrestler, weighing in at 95 kg, is training on a cycle at 175 Watts. Find absolute $\dot{V}O_2$, relative $\dot{V}O_2$, and METs.

9. Bill, who weighs 120 kg, is riding a cycle at 200 Watts. Find METs and kcal/min. Approximately how many kcal will Bill expend riding the cycle for 20 min? If this problem will not work out for you, carefully write out all of the units for each section of the problem, making sure that all units cancel appropriately.

10. An exercise prescription for Mr. Mack, who weighs 100 kg, recommends that he train on a cycle ergometer at a level of 7 METs. What workload in kgm/min should be used? (Remember: Subtract and invert.)

11. On a maximal TM GXT, a 95-kg subject achieved 15 METs. Prescribe a cycle workload in kgm/min that is 80% of the 15 METs.

12. Find cycle resistance in kg from the following information. Make sure that all units cancel except the kg.

$$\frac{1{,}010 \text{ kg m}}{\text{min}} \qquad \frac{6 \text{ m}}{\text{rev}} \qquad \frac{80 \text{ rev}}{\text{min}}$$

13. A 176-lb man reaches 12 METs on a maximal cycle GXT. The exercise prescription suggests that he train at 70% of max effort. Determine

    (a) $\frac{\text{kgm}}{\text{min}}$ workload

    (b) Watts

    (c) pedaling resistance in kg, at 6 m/rev and 80 rev/min

14. Given 1,200 kgm/min, weight of subject = 95 kg, and cycling rate = 50 rev/min, find total $\dot{V}O_2$ and METs.

15. Given 10 METs and subject's weight of 80 kg, find kgm/min and Watts.

Practice problems 16 through 24 deal exclusively with arm ergometry. While performing these problems, think *arm ergometer, small muscle groups.*

16. For the arm ergometer equation, determine the resting $\dot{V}O_2$ component for each of the following subjects. Write out all of the units.

    (a) Subject's wt = 65 kg

    (b) wt = 145 lbs

17. Determine the resistive $\dot{V}O_2$ component for the arm ergometer equation for each of the following. Write out the units.

    (a) 150 kgm/min

    (b) 225 $\frac{\text{kgm}}{\text{min}}$

18. Convert the following absolute $\dot{V}O_2$ values into relative $\dot{V}O_2$ values.

    (a) 425 ml O_2/min wt = 62 kg

    (b) 1,920 ml O_2/min wt = 165 lb

19. Given the following information for the arm ergometer, determine the total $\dot{V}O_2$. Hint: Use Total $\dot{V}O_2$ = resistive $\dot{V}O_2$ + rest $\dot{V}O_2$.

    (a) Workload = 625 kgm/min and wt = 92 kg

    (b) wt = 70 kg and workload = 700 kgm/min

20. Given the following information for the arm ergometer, determine workloads in the units of kgm/min. Hint: First subtract the resting $\dot{V}O_2$ from the total $\dot{V}O_2$.

    (a) wt = 60 kg Total $\dot{V}O_2$ = 1,825 ml O_2/min

    (b) wt = 78 kg Total $\dot{V}O_2$ = 1,325 ml O_2/min

21. Convert the following into Watts. Write out each problem.

    (a) 538 kgm/min

    (b) $\frac{350 \text{ kgm}}{\text{min}}$

22. Convert the following into kgm/min.

    (a) 125 Watts

    (b) 75 Watts

23. Find workload using the equation:

$$\text{Workload (kgm/min)} = \frac{\text{kg}}{1} \times \frac{6\ \text{m}}{\text{rev}} \times \frac{60\ \text{rev}}{\text{min}}$$

To help you remember, write out the equation for each problem.

(a) 1.5 kg

(b) .80 kg

24. Determine kg of arm cranking resistance.

Use this equation: $\text{kg} = \frac{\text{kgm}}{\text{min}} \times \frac{\text{rev}}{\text{m}} \times \frac{\text{min}}{\text{rev}}$

Write out the equation for each of the problems. Make sure that all of the units cancel out appropriately.

(a) $\frac{540\ \text{kgm}}{\text{min}} \quad \frac{\text{rev}}{6\ \text{m}} \quad \frac{\text{min}}{60\ \text{rev}}$

(b) $\frac{270\ \text{kgm}}{\text{min}} \quad \frac{6\ \text{m}}{\text{rev}} \quad \frac{\text{min}}{60\ \text{rev}}$

(c) $\frac{720\ \text{kgm}}{\text{min}} \quad \frac{6\ \text{m}}{\text{rev}} \quad \frac{60\ \text{rev}}{\text{min}}$

25. Use Table 10.1. Holly is pedaling a Monark cycle at 90 rev/min (rpm) with a resistance setting of 4 kg. Determine workload in the units kgm/min.

26. Use Table 10.1. David is pedaling a Tunturi cycle at 100 rev/min. The resistance is set on 2 kg. What is the workload in Watts and kgm/min?

27. David's body weight is 75 kg. Use Table 10.2 to find his MET level.

28. We want Jane to train at 200 Watts of workload on the Monark cycle. What are two possible workload settings that will achieve this objective? Use Table 10.1.

For questions 29 and 30, if at first your answers do not seem to be correct, try to work the problem in different ways before you look at the answers.

Remember, when solving for total $\dot{V}O_2$, resting $\dot{V}O_2$ is *added.* When solving for workload, the rest $\dot{V}O_2$ must first be *subtracted.*

29. Chris, who weighs 68 kg, is working out on a cycle pedaling at a total absolute $\dot{V}O_2$ of 3,500 ml O_2/min. Determine her workload at this $\dot{V}O_2$.

30. Jonathan, who weighs 165 lb, reaches 15 METs on a maximal cycle test. We are certain that his effort was a true $\dot{V}O_2$max because O_2 uptake, as measured with an O_2 analyzer and open-circuit spirometry, began to level off near the time of exhaustion; his R value was at 1.11. His exercise prescription calls for 80% of $\dot{V}O_2$max using 80 rev/min as a pedaling speed.

Find (a) kgm/min, (b) Watts, (c) kg of pedal resistance, and (d) kcal expenditure at the 80%.

Chapter 10 Answers to Practice Problems

1. (a) 63.64 kg

(b) 84.09 kg

2. (a) 202.40 lb

   (b) 143 lb

Answers 3 through 15 relate to the cycle ergometer.

3. $$\text{Absolute } \dot{V}O_2 = \left(\frac{1{,}500\ \cancel{\text{kgm}}}{\text{min}} \times \frac{2\ \text{ml } O_2}{\cancel{\text{kgm}}}\right) + \left(\frac{3.5\ \text{ml } O_2}{\cancel{\text{kg}}/\text{min}} \times \frac{84\ \cancel{\text{kg}}}{1}\right)$$

$$\text{Absolute } \dot{V}O_2 = \frac{3{,}000\ \text{ml } O_2}{\text{min}} + \frac{294\ \text{ml } O_2}{\text{min}}$$

$$\text{Absolute } \dot{V}O_2 = \frac{3{,}294\ \text{ml } O_2}{\text{min}}$$

$$\text{Relative } \dot{V}O_2 = \frac{3{,}294\ \text{ml } O_2/\text{min}}{84\ \text{kg}} = 39.21\ \text{ml } O_2/\text{kg/min}$$

Converting to METs:

$$39.21\ \cancel{\text{ml } O_2/\text{kg/min}} \times \frac{1\ \text{MET}}{3.5\ \cancel{\text{ml } O_2/\text{kg/min}}} = 11.2\ \text{METs}$$

4. Absolute $\dot{V}O_2$ = 2,980 ml O_2/min or 10.64 METs (2,980/80 = 37.25)

   This subject is expending about 15 kcal/min, i.e.,

$$\frac{2{,}980\ \cancel{\text{ml } O_2}}{\text{min}} \times \frac{.005\ \text{kcal}}{\cancel{\text{ml } O_2}} = \frac{14.9\ \text{kcal}}{\text{min}}.$$

5. $$\frac{1{,}890\ \text{ml } O_2/\text{min}}{105\ \text{kg}} = 18\ \text{ml } O_2/\text{kg/min}$$

$$18\ \cancel{\text{ml } O_2/\text{kg/min}} \times \frac{1\ \text{MET}}{3.5\ \cancel{\text{ml } O_2/\text{kg/min}}} = 5.14\ \text{METs}$$

6. 5.08 METs

7. $$\frac{1{,}869\ \cancel{\text{ml } O_2}}{\text{min}} \times \frac{.005\ \text{kcal}}{\cancel{\text{ml } O_2}} = \frac{9.345\ \text{kcal}}{\text{min}}, \text{ almost } \frac{10\ \text{kcal}}{\text{min}}$$

   The kcal conversion factor is the one you'll tend to forget during the pressure of an exam. Remember, it is .005 kcal on the top, i.e., .005 kcal/ml O_2.

8. Absolute $\dot{V}O_2$ = 2,432.50 ml O_2/min
   Relative $\dot{V}O_2$ = 25.61 ml O_2/kg/min and approximately 7.32 METs

9. 6.71 METs and 14.1 kcal/min (approximately 282 kcal expended in 20 min)

10. Solving for workload

    Step 1: Convert METs to relative $\dot{V}O_2$.

$$7\ \cancel{\text{METs}} \times \frac{3.5\ \text{ml } O_2/\text{kg/min}}{1\ \cancel{\text{MET}}} = 24.5\ \text{ml } O_2/\text{kg/min}$$

$$\frac{24.5\ \text{ml } O_2}{\cancel{\text{kg}}/\text{min}} \times 100\ \cancel{\text{kg}} = \frac{2450\ \text{ml } O_2}{\text{min}} = \text{total } \dot{V}O_2$$

    Step 2: Calculate the absolute resting $\dot{V}O_2$.

$$\text{Rest } \dot{V}O_2 = \overset{\text{(Relative)}}{\frac{3.5 \text{ ml } O_2}{\cancel{\text{kg}}/\text{min}}} \times 100 \cancel{\text{ kg}} = \overset{\text{(Absolute)}}{\frac{350 \text{ ml } O_2}{\text{min}}}$$

Step 3: Subtract the resting $\dot{V}O_2$ from the total $\dot{V}O_2$.

$$\begin{array}{lrl} \text{Total } \dot{V}O_2 = & & 2{,}450 \text{ ml } O_2/\text{min} \\ \text{Rest } \dot{V}O_2 = & - & 350 \text{ ml } O_2/\text{min} \\ \hline & & 2{,}100 \text{ ml } O_2/\text{min} = \text{resistive } \dot{V}O_2 \end{array}$$

Step 4: Invert the 2 ml O_2/kgm and multiply.

$$\frac{2{,}100 \cancel{\text{ ml } O_2}}{\text{min}} \times \frac{\text{kgm}}{2 \cancel{\text{ ml } O_2}} = \frac{1{,}050 \text{ kgm}}{\text{min}}$$

11. First take 80% of the max achieved METs. Math check follows.

    Step 1: 15 METs × .80 = 12 METs = 42 ml O_2/kg/min

    Step 2: $\frac{42 \text{ ml } O_2}{\cancel{\text{kg}}/\text{min}} \times 95 \cancel{\text{ kg}} = 3{,}990 \text{ ml } O_2/\text{min}$

    Step 3: $\frac{3.5 \text{ ml } O_2}{\cancel{\text{kg}}/\text{min}} \times 95 \cancel{\text{ kg}} = 332.5 \text{ ml } O_2/\text{min}$

    Step 4: 3,990 ml O_2/min − 332.5 ml O_2/min = 3,657.5 ml O_2/min

    Step 5: Rearrange the cycle equation.

    $$\frac{3{,}657.5 \cancel{\text{ ml } O_2}}{\text{min}} \times \frac{\text{kgm}}{2 \cancel{\text{ ml } O_2}} = 1{,}828.75 \text{ kgm/min (about 300 Watts)}$$

12. $\frac{1{,}010 \text{ kg} \cancel{\text{ m}}}{\cancel{\text{min}}} \times \frac{\cancel{\text{rev}}}{6 \cancel{\text{ m}}} \times \frac{\cancel{\text{min}}}{80 \cancel{\text{ rev}}} = 2.1 \text{ kg of pedal resistance}$

13. Check list: 80-kg man
    70% = 8.4 METs
    absolute $\dot{V}O_2$ = 2,352 ml O_2/min
    2,352 ml O_2/min − 280 ml O_2/min = 2,072 ml O_2/min

    (a) $\frac{1{,}036 \text{ kgm}}{\text{min}}$ (b) 172.67 Watts (c) 2.16 kg of pedaling resistance

14. 2,732.5 ml O_2/min

    28.76 ml O_2/kg/min = 8.22 METs

    Round off your final answer of METs to two decimal places.

15. $\frac{1{,}260 \text{ kgm}}{\text{min}} = 210 \text{ Watts}$

16. (a) 227.50 ml O_2/min

    (b) 145 lb = 66 kg, 230.68 ml O_2/min

17. (a) 450 ml O_2/min

    (b) 675 ml O_2/min

18. (a) 6.85 ml O_2/kg/min

    (b) 165 lb = 75 kg, 25.60 ml O_2/kg/min

19. Total absolute $\dot{V}O_2$ for arm ergometer

    (a) 2,197 ml O_2/min

    (b) 2,345 ml O_2/min

20. (a)

$$\begin{array}{lrr} \text{Total } \dot{V}O_2 = & & 1{,}825 \text{ ml } O_2/\text{min} \\ \text{Rest } \dot{V}O_2 = & - & 210 \text{ ml } O_2/\text{min} \\ \hline & & 1{,}615 \text{ ml } O_2/\text{min} \end{array}$$

$$\frac{1{,}615 \cancel{\text{ml } O_2}}{\text{min}} \times \frac{\text{kgm}}{3 \cancel{\text{ml } O_2}} = \frac{538.33 \text{ kgm}}{\text{min}}$$

    (b) 350.67 kgm/min

21. (a) $538 \cancel{\text{kgm/min}} \times \dfrac{1 \text{ Watt}}{6 \cancel{\text{kgm/min}}} = 89.67 \text{ Watts}$

    (b) 58.33 Watts

22. (a) 750 kgm/min

    (b) 450 kgm/min

23. (a) 540 kgm/min

    (b) 288 kgm/min

24. (a) 1.5 kg of cranking resistance on the Monark arm ergometer

    (b) .75 kg

    (c) 2.0 kg

25. 2,160 kgm/min and 360 Watts

26. 200 Watts and 1,200 kgm/min

27. 10.6 METs (1,200 kgm/min and 75 kg of body weight)

    Note: Pedaling at 100 rev/min and 2 kg is the same as 50 rev/min and 4 kg of resistance.

28. 100 rev/min and 2 kg; 50 rev/min and 4 kg

29. Solving for workload: You are given the total $\dot{V}O_2$ as 3,500 ml O_2/min and must determine the cycle workload in kgm/min. Wt = 68 kg.

    This is how the equation would look. The ? is the unknown workload.

$$3{,}500 \text{ ml } O_2/\text{min} = \left(\frac{? \text{ kgm}}{\text{min}} \times \frac{2 \text{ ml } O_2}{\text{kgm}}\right) + \left(\frac{3.5 \text{ ml } O_2}{\text{kg/min}} \times 68 \text{ kg}\right)$$

    Step 1: Convert the resting $\dot{V}O_2$ to an absolute $\dot{V}O_2$.

$$\frac{3.5 \text{ ml } O_2}{\cancel{\text{kg}}/\text{min}} \times 68 \cancel{\text{kg}} = 238 \text{ ml } O_2/\text{min}$$

    Step 2: Subtract the resting $\dot{V}O_2$ from the total $\dot{V}O_2$.

$$\begin{array}{lrr} \text{Total } \dot{V}O_2 = & & 3{,}500 \text{ ml } O_2/\text{min} \\ \text{Rest } \dot{V}O_2 = & - & 238 \text{ ml } O_2/\text{min} \\ \hline & & 3{,}262 \text{ ml } O_2/\text{min} \end{array}$$

Step 3: Now the equation will look like this (the resistive $\dot{V}O_2$ component of the cycle equation).

$$\frac{3{,}262 \text{ ml } O_2}{\text{min}} = \frac{? \text{ kgm}}{\text{min}} \times \frac{2 \text{ ml } O_2}{\text{kgm}}$$

Step 4: Invert the 2 ml $O_2$2/kgm and multiply.

$$\frac{3{,}262 \cancel{\text{ml } O_2}}{\text{min}} \times \frac{\text{kgm}}{2 \cancel{\text{ml } O_2}} = \frac{1{,}631 \text{ kgm}}{\text{min}}$$

Remember, when given the total $\dot{V}O_2$, subtract, invert, and multiply. The 1,631 kgm/min would be the workload at a total VO_2 of 3,500 ml O_2/min.

Step 5: Convert 1,631 kgm/min to Watts.

$$1{,}631 \cancel{\text{kgm/min}} \times \frac{1 \text{ Watt}}{6 \cancel{\text{kgm/min}}} = 271.83 \text{ Watts}$$

(See Table 10.1. At 50 rev/min the 271 Watts would be a kg setting between the 5 kg and 6 kg. At 90 rev/min this would be 3 kg.)

Extra information

Let's say an exercise prescription suggests that our subject train at 80% of $\dot{V}O_2$max. We could have used 80% of the original 3,500 ml O_2/min, i.e. 3,500(.80) = 2,800 ml O_2/min, using this number as the total $\dot{V}O_2$ throughout the problem.

The other option would be to use 80% of the final answer of 271 Watts (80% of 271 Watts equals 216.8 Watts, rounded off to 217 Watts). The 217 Watts would then be used as the exercise prescription for the cycle ergometer. At 217 Watts (see Table 10.1) our subject could train at

(a) 100 rev/min and 2 kg, or

(b) 70 rev/min and 3 kg, or

(c) about 50 rev/min and 4 kg of pedaling resistance.

30. For a 165-lb man, max effort = 15 METs. You are finding kgm/min, Watts, kg of pedaling resistance, and kcal/min at 80% of $\dot{V}O_2$max. As you read through this answer, use a pencil to cancel the appropriate units.

Step 1: Convert lb of body wt to kg.

$$165 \cancel{\text{lb}} \times \frac{1 \text{ kg}}{2.2 \cancel{\text{kg}}} = 75 \text{ kg}$$

Step 2: Determine 80% of the $\dot{V}O_2$max.

$$15 \text{ METs}(.80) = 12 \text{ METs}$$

Step 3: Convert the METs to a relative $\dot{V}O_2$.

$$12 \cancel{\text{METs}} \times \frac{3.5 \text{ ml } O_2/\text{kg/min}}{1 \cancel{\text{MET}}} = 42 \text{ ml } O_2/\text{kg/min}$$

Step 4: Convert the total relative $\dot{V}O_2$ to an absolute $\dot{V}O_2$ by using the subject's weight.

$$\frac{42 \text{ ml } O_2}{\cancel{\text{kg}}/\text{min}} \times 75 \cancel{\text{kg}} = \frac{3{,}150 \text{ ml } O_2}{\text{min}}$$

Step 5: Set up the entire cycle equation.

$$\underset{(\text{Total } \dot{V}O_2)}{\frac{3{,}150 \text{ ml } O_2}{\text{min}}} = \underset{(\text{Resistive } \dot{V}O_2)}{\left(\frac{? \text{ kgm}}{\text{min}} \times \frac{2 \text{ ml } O_2}{\text{kgm}}\right)} + \underset{(\text{Rest } \dot{V}O_2)}{\left(\frac{3.5 \text{ ml } O_2}{\text{kg}/\text{min}} \times 75 \text{ kg}\right)}$$

Step 6: Determine resting $\dot{V}O_2$ (ml O_2/min).

$$\frac{3.5 \text{ ml } O_2}{\cancel{\text{kg}}/\text{min}} \times 75 \cancel{\text{kg}} = \frac{262.5 \text{ ml } O_2}{\text{min}}$$

Now we can subtract numbers with like units.

Step 7: Subtract the rest $\dot{V}O_2$ from the total $\dot{V}O_2$.

$$\begin{array}{lcr} \text{Total } \dot{V}O_2 & = & 3{,}150.0 \text{ ml } O_2/\text{min} \\ \text{Rest } \dot{V}O_2 & = & -\ \ 262.5 \text{ ml } O_2/\text{min} \\ \hline & & 2{,}887.5 \text{ ml } O_2/\text{min} \end{array} = \text{resistive } \dot{V}O_2 \text{ component}$$

Step 8: With the resting $\dot{V}O_2$ eliminated, the resistive component now looks like this:

$$\frac{2{,}887.5 \text{ ml } O_2}{\text{min}} = \frac{? \text{ kgm}}{\text{min}} \times \frac{2 \text{ ml } O_2}{\text{kgm}}$$

Step 9: Invert $\frac{2 \text{ ml } O_2}{\text{kgm}}$ and multiply.

$$\frac{2{,}887.5 \cancel{\text{ml } O_2}}{\text{min}} \times \frac{\text{kgm}}{2 \cancel{\text{ml } O_2}} = \frac{1{,}443.75 \text{ kgm}}{\text{min}} = \text{answer (a).}$$

Step 10: Convert kgm/min to Watts.

$$1{,}443.75 \cancel{\text{kgm/min}} \times \frac{1 \text{ Watt}}{6 \cancel{\text{kgm/min}}} = 240.63 \text{ Watts} = \text{answer (b).}$$

Step 11: Determine kg of pedaling resistance.

$$\frac{1{,}443.75 \text{ kg } \cancel{\text{m}}}{\cancel{\text{min}}} \times \frac{1 \cancel{\text{rev}}}{6 \cancel{\text{m}}} \times \frac{1 \cancel{\text{min}}}{80 \cancel{\text{rev}}} = \text{approx 3 kg of pedal resistance,}$$

which is answer (c).

Check answers (a), (b), and (c) with Table 10.1.

Now determine the energy expenditure in kcal/min of this subject at his 80% of $\dot{V}O_2$max.
Use the absolute $\dot{V}O_2$ value of 3,150 ml O_2/min.

$$\frac{3{,}150 \cancel{\text{ml } O_2}}{\text{min}} \times \frac{.005 \text{ kcal}}{\cancel{\text{ml } O_2}} = \frac{15.75 \text{ kcal}}{\text{min}}, \text{ which is answer (d).}$$

11 Calculations for Bench Stepping

Major Concepts

Calculating workload for bench stepping

The bench stepping equation

Solving the ACSM bench stepping equation for total $\dot{V}O_2$

Solving for horizontal and vertical $\dot{V}O_2$

Solving for step height, steps/min, and kcal/min

A bench step is the most inexpensive and simplest ergometer for exercise testing and training. The stepping bench is also an excellent mode for field submaximal fitness testing as outlined in chapter 12. As you progress through the example and practice problems, compare your answers with the $\dot{V}O_2$ values presented in Table 11.1, a quick reference table.

Table 11.2 provides an outline of the advantages and disadvantages of using a bench for exercise training and exercise testing.

Calculating Stepping Workload

In bench stepping, the workload (resistance) is based on body weight, stepping rate, and step height. For the cycle or arm ergometer, workload is based on pedal speed and pedal resistance, whereas treadmill workload is a function of speed, grade, and body weight.

The amount of work performed in one cycle of stepping can be calculated from the work equation:

$$\text{Work} = \text{force (body weight)} \times \text{distance (step height)}$$

Table 11.1 Total $\dot{V}O_2$ Values (ml O_2/kg/min) Based upon Height of Step and Rate of Stepping using Bench Stepping Equation (ACSM, 1995).

(Step height) Inches	Meters	16 / 64	20 / 80	24 / 96	28 / 112	32 / 128	36 / 144	40 / 160	Step/min Clicks/min (metronome)
6	0.154	11.51	14.39	17.27	20.15	23.03	25.91	28.78	
8	0.203	13.40	16.74	20.10	23.44	26.79	30.14	33.49	
10	0.254	15.35	19.19	23.03	26.87	30.70	34.55	38.38	
12	0.305	17.31	21.64	25.97	30.30	34.62	38.95	43.28	
14	0.356	19.24	24.09	28.91	33.72	38.54	43.36	48.18	
16	0.406	21.19	26.49	31.79	37.08	42.38	47.68	52.98	
18	0.457	23.15	28.94	34.72	40.51	46.30	52.08	57.87	
20	0.508	25.11	31.38	37.66	43.94	50.21	56.49	62.77	
22	0.559	27.07	33.83	40.60	47.36	54.13	60.90	67.66	

Divide $\dot{V}O_2$ values by 3.5 ml O_2/kg/min to solve for METs.

The work of one cycle is multiplied by the step rate (cycles/min) to determine total work. The work of stepping down is usually ignored. The following example illustrates the calculation of workload.

Example 11A

Solve for bench stepping workload. An 80-kg man stepped up and down on an 8-in bench at the rate of 25 steps per minute. What was his workload per minute?

Step 1: Convert inches to meters.

$$8 \text{ in} \times \frac{1 \text{ m}}{39.37 \text{ in}} = .203 \text{ m}$$

Step 2: Work out the equation and substitute known values.

$$\begin{aligned} \text{Workload} &= \text{force (body wt [kg])} \times \text{distance (step ht [m/step])} \\ &\quad \times \text{step rate (step/min)} \\ &= \frac{80 \text{ kg}}{1} \times \frac{.203 \text{ m}}{\cancel{\text{step}}} \times \frac{25 \cancel{\text{step}}}{\text{min}} \\ &= 406 \frac{\text{kgm}}{\text{min}} \end{aligned}$$

Calculating Step Rate to Achieve a Desired Workload

Many times you are provided an exercise prescription requiring a specific workload. Your facility has one bench of a specific height. Example 11B illustrates how you can determine the step rate necessary to achieve the desired workload.

Table 11.2 Advantages and Disadvantages of Exercise Testing With a Stepping Bench

Advantages
(a) Simple design, low cost, and easy construction; low cost if purchased from a vendor.
(b) Multipurpose; a bench from a bench aerobics class can be used for training or exercise testing.
(c) Low maintenance.
(d) No calibration required.
(e) Easily stored
(f) No electrical components; does not have to be plugged in.
(g) Movement pattern familiar and easy to learn.
(h) An excellent mode for submaximal exercise testing.
Disadvantages
(a) Not well suited for maximal effort testing. Subjects, in general, are not able to reach physiological upper limits while stepping.
(b) It is difficult or impossible to record pulse and BP while a subject is stepping.
(c) Different step heights are necessary as dictated by the population undergoing submaximal testing or for exercise training.
(d) Stepping becomes hazardous at stepping rates above 45 cycles per minute. Four footsteps (up and down once) is one cycle.
(e) Subjects may fall or trip over the step and a hand, wrist, face, or neck injury can result.

Example 11B

Solve for stepping rate. Jim, an 80-kg man, would like to exercise at 600 kgm/min on a 12-in (.305 m) step. What step rate would achieve this workload?

Step 1: Write out equation and substitute known values.

Workload (kgm/min) = force (body wt [kg]) × distance (step ht [m/step]) × step rate (step/min)

$$600\,\frac{\text{kgm}}{\text{min}} = \frac{80\text{ kg}}{1} \times \frac{.305\text{ m}}{\text{step}} \times \text{step rate}\left(\frac{\text{step}}{\text{min}}\right)$$

Step 2: Perform the math.

$$600\,\frac{\text{kgm}}{\text{min}} = \frac{24.4\text{ kgm}}{\text{step}} \times \text{step rate}\left(\frac{\text{step}}{\text{min}}\right)$$

Step 3: Invert 24.4 kgm/step and multiply.

$$\frac{600\text{ }\cancel{\text{kgm}}}{\text{min}} \times \frac{\text{step}}{24.4\text{ }\cancel{\text{kgm}}} = \text{approximately } 25\,\frac{\text{steps}}{\text{min}}$$

To achieve a step rate of 25 steps/min, set the metronome at 100 clicks per minute, i.e.,

4 steps per cycle × 25 cycles = 100 foot plants or 100 metro clicks/min

The equation used in Example 11B can also be used to find the proper step height to achieve a desired workload if you know the step rate and the subject's body weight.

Calculating $\dot{V}O_2$ During Bench Stepping

The ACSM (1995) bench step equation is the most popular equation for estimating steady-state oxygen consumption relative to body weight (ml O_2/kg/min). The ACSM equation involves both a horizontal and vertical component that are combined to calculate total $\dot{V}O_2$.

$$\text{Horizontal } \dot{V}O_2 = \text{step rate}\left(\frac{\text{step}}{\text{min}}\right) \times \frac{.35 \text{ ml } O_2/\text{kg/min}}{\text{step/min}}$$

$$\text{Vertical } \dot{V}O_2 = \text{step height}\left(\frac{\text{m}}{\text{step}}\right) \times \text{step rate}\left(\frac{\text{step}}{\text{min}}\right) \times \frac{2.4 \text{ ml } O_2/\text{kg/min}}{\text{m/min}}$$

$$\text{Total } \dot{V}O_2 = \text{horizontal } \dot{V}O_2 + \text{vertical } \dot{V}O_2 \text{ (ml } O_2/\text{kg/min)}$$

where:

a) Step rate is the number of stepping cycles (up and down) per minute (included in both horizontal and vertical components);
b) 0.35 ml O_2/kg/min is the oxygen cost of stepping back and forth along the horizontal plane in 1 min;
c) step height (m/step) is the height of the step in meters;
d) 2.4 ml O_2/kg/min is the oxygen cost of stepping up and down per meter per min (stepping up [positive = 1.8 ml O_2/kg/min/m/min] and down [negative = .6 ml O_2/kg/min/m/min]).

The vert $\dot{V}O_2$ component is always going to be a much larger number than the horiz $\dot{V}O_2$. In the vert $\dot{V}O_2$ component, a subject lifts his or her entire body weight almost straight up and down, requiring much more O_2, while the horizontal component requires only minimal O_2 cost to move parallel to the pull of gravity.

The following examples illustrate calculation of total $\dot{V}O_2$, step height, step rate, and other elements of bench stepping. In some of the examples the units have been canceled as an illustration. In others, units have not been canceled. As you work through the examples cancel the appropriate units to make sure you are correct.

Example 11C

Use the bench step equation to solve for total $\dot{V}O_2$. Caleb is stepping at 30 steps/min on a step .46 m high. Find his total $\dot{V}O_2$ and METs.

Step 1: Solve the horizontal component.

$$\text{Horiz } \dot{V}O_2 = \frac{30 \text{ step}}{\text{min}} \times \frac{0.35 \text{ ml } O_2/\text{kg/min}}{\text{step/min}}$$

$$\text{Horiz } \dot{V}O_2 = 10.5 \frac{\text{ml } O_2}{\text{kg/min}}, \text{ also written } 10.5 \text{ ml } O_2/\text{kg/min}$$

Step 2: Solve the vertical component.

$$\text{Vert } \dot{V}O_2 = \frac{.46\ \cancel{m}}{\cancel{step}} \times \frac{30\ \cancel{step}}{\cancel{min}} \times \frac{2.4\ ml\ O_2/kg/\cancel{min}}{\cancel{m}/min}$$
$$\text{Vert } \dot{V}O_2 = 33.12\ ml\ O_2/kg/min$$

Step 3: Add the horiz $\dot{V}O_2$ to the vert $\dot{V}O_2$.

$$\begin{aligned} \text{Horiz } \dot{V}O_2 &= \quad 10.50\ ml\ O_2/kg/min \\ \text{Vert } \dot{V}O_2 &= \underline{+\ 33.12\ ml\ O_2/kg/min} \\ & \quad\ \ 43.62\ ml\ O_2/kg/min = \text{total } \dot{V}O_2 \end{aligned}$$

Step 4: Convert the total $\dot{V}O_2$ into METs

$$43.62\ \cancel{ml\ O_2/kg/min} \times \frac{1\ MET}{3.5\ \cancel{ml\ O_2/kg/min}} = 12.46\ METs$$

Example 11D

Solve for the horiz and vert $\dot{V}O_2$. Carol, who has a total $\dot{V}O_2$ of 44.5 ml O_2/kg/min, is stepping at a rate of 30 steps/min. Find her horiz $\dot{V}O_2$ and vert $\dot{V}O_2$.

Step 1: Solve for horiz $\dot{V}O_2$.

$$\text{Horiz } \dot{V}O_2 = \frac{30\ step}{min} \times \frac{0.35\ ml\ O_2/kg/min}{step/min}$$
$$\text{Horiz } \dot{V}O_2 = 10.5\ ml\ O_2/kg/min$$

Step 2: Find vert $\dot{V}O_2$ by subtracting horiz from total $\dot{V}O_2$.

$$\begin{aligned} &(\text{Total } \dot{V}O_2) && - (\text{horiz } \dot{V}O_2) && = (\text{vert } \dot{V}O_2) \\ &44.5\ ml\ O_2/kg/min && - 10.5\ ml\ O_2/kg/min && = 34\ ml\ O_2/kg/min \end{aligned}$$

Example 11E

Solve for height of the step. Now that we know the value for the vert $\dot{V}O_2$ from Example 11D, we can solve for height (m) of the step.

Step 1: Write out the vert $\dot{V}O_2$ component from the stepping equation. Multiply 30 times 2.4 and cancel the units.

$$34\ ml\ O_2/kg/min = \frac{30\ step}{\cancel{min}} \times \frac{2.4\ ml\ O_2/kg/\cancel{min}}{m/min} \times \frac{?\ m}{step}$$

$$34\ ml\ O_2/kg/min = \frac{72\ ml\ O_2/kg \times step}{m/min} \times \frac{?\ m}{step}$$

Step 2: Rearrange, invert, cancel, and multiply. As you practice this process a few times, you will see that it is easy and straightforward.

$$34\ \cancel{ml\ O_2/kg/min} \times \frac{m/\cancel{min}}{72\ \cancel{ml\ O_2/kg} \times step} = \frac{.472\ m}{step}$$

Example 11F

Solve for vert $\dot{V}O_2$. Given a step height of .457 m/step and a stepping rate of 30 step/min, find vertical $\dot{V}O_2$.

Step 1: Enter the given values into the vert $\dot{V}O_2$ component. Cancel the appropriate units and multiply.

$$\text{Vert } \dot{V}O_2 = \frac{.46\ \cancel{\text{m}}}{\cancel{\text{step}}} \times \frac{30\ \cancel{\text{step}}}{\cancel{\text{min}}} \times \frac{2.4\ \text{ml } O_2/\text{kg}/\cancel{\text{min}}}{\cancel{\text{m}}/\text{min}}$$

$$\text{Vert } \dot{V}O_2 = 33.12\ \text{ml } O_2/\text{kg}/\text{min}$$

To get an idea how high .457 meters is you can convert the meters to inches, as follows.

$$.457\ \cancel{\text{m}} \times \frac{39.27\ \text{in}}{1\ \cancel{\text{m}}} = 18\ \text{in}$$

A 20-inch step is the standard height for the Harvard step test. In the bench step equation the unit m (meters) will always be used rather than the unit inches. The YMCA step test uses a 12-in step.

Example 11G

Solve for m/step in the vert $\dot{V}O_2$ component. Given a vert $\dot{V}O_2$ of 33.12 ml O_2/kg/min and a stepping rate of 30 step/min, find m/step.

Step 1: Enter the values into the vert $\dot{V}O_2$ component.

$$\frac{33.12\ \text{ml } O_2/\text{kg}}{\text{min}} = \frac{?\ \text{m}}{\text{step}} \times \frac{30\ \text{step}}{\cancel{\text{min}}} \times \frac{2.4\ \text{ml } O_2/\text{kg}/\cancel{\text{min}}}{\text{m}/\text{min}}$$

$$\frac{33.12\ \text{ml } O_2/\text{kg}}{\text{min}} = \frac{?\ \text{m}}{\text{step}} \times \frac{72\ \text{ml } O_2/\text{kg} \times \text{step}}{\text{m}/\text{min}}$$

Step 2: Rearrange the equation, invert, cancel, and multiply.

$$\frac{33.12\ \cancel{\text{ml } O_2/\text{kg}}}{\cancel{\text{min}}} \times \frac{\text{m}/\cancel{\text{min}}}{72\ \cancel{\text{ml } O_2/\text{kg}} \times \text{step}} = \frac{.46\ \text{m}}{\text{step}}$$

Example 11H

Solve for kcal/min of energy expenditure. From Example 11C, we know that Caleb (who weighs 72 kg) has a total $\dot{V}O_2$ of 43.62 ml O_2/kg/min. Find how many kcal/min Caleb would be expending during his stepping.

Step 1: Convert the total (relative) $\dot{V}O_2$ into a total (absolute) $\dot{V}O_2$.

(Relative) (Absolute)

$$\frac{43.62\ \text{ml } O_2}{\cancel{\text{kg}}/\text{min}} \times \frac{72\ \cancel{\text{kg}}}{1} = \frac{3{,}140.64\ \text{ml } O_2}{\text{min}}$$

Step 2: Determine kcal/min. Use .005 kcal/ml O_2 as the conversion factor.

$$\frac{3{,}140.64\ \cancel{\text{ml } O_2}}{\text{min}} \times \frac{.005\ \text{kcal}}{\cancel{\text{ml } O_2}} = \frac{15.70\ \text{kcal}}{\text{min}}$$

At a stepping rate of 30 step/min using a .46-m bench, Caleb has a total $\dot{V}O_2$ of 43.62 ml O_2/kg/min and is expending energy at a rate of almost 16 kcal/min.

Example 11I

Solve for step/min using the whole bench step equation. Edward achieved a $\dot{V}O_2$max of 53 ml O_2/kg/min on a GXT. His exercise prescription suggested that he train at 85% of his $\dot{V}O_2$max: 53 ml O_2/kg/min × .85 = 45 ml O_2/kg/min.

You have one bench in your fitness center that is .5 m high. You need to determine the correct stepping rate to satisfy the exercise prescription.

Step 1: Enter the given values into the bench step equation and multiply.

$$45 \text{ ml } O_2/\text{kg/min} =$$

$$\left(\frac{?\text{ step}}{\text{min}} \times \frac{0.35 \text{ ml } O_2/\text{kg/min}}{\text{step/min}}\right) + \left(\frac{?\text{ step}}{\text{min}} \times \frac{.5 \text{ m}}{\text{step}} \times \frac{2.4 \text{ ml } O_2/\text{kg/min}}{\text{m/min}}\right)$$

$$45 \text{ ml } O_2/\text{kg/min} =$$

$$\left(\frac{?\text{ step}}{\text{min}} \times \frac{0.35 \text{ ml } O_2/\text{kg/min}}{\text{step/min}}\right) + \left(\frac{?\text{ step}}{\text{min}} \times \frac{1.2 \text{ ml } O_2/\text{kg/min}}{\text{step/min}}\right)$$

Step 2: Add the like terms.

$$45 \text{ ml } O_2/\text{kg/min} = \left(\frac{?\text{ step}}{\text{min}} \times 0.35\right) + \left(\frac{?\text{ step}}{\text{min}} \times 1.2\right)$$

to

$$= \frac{?\text{ step}}{\text{min}} \times (0.35 + 1.2)$$

$$= \frac{?\text{ step}}{\text{min}} \times \frac{1.55 \text{ ml } O_2/\text{kg/min}}{\text{step/min}}$$

$$45 \text{ ml } O_2/\text{kg/min} = \frac{?\text{ step}}{\text{min}} \times \frac{1.55 \text{ ml } O_2/\text{kg/min}}{\text{step/min}}$$

Because their units are the same, the 0.35 and the 1.2 can be added.

Step 3: To solve for step/min we must isolate the step/min to one side of the equation, invert the 1.55 with the units, cancel, and multiply.

$$45 \cancel{\text{ml } O_2/\text{kg/min}} \times \frac{\text{step/min}}{1.55 \cancel{\text{ml } O_2/\text{kg/min}}} = \text{step/min}$$

$$29 \text{ step/min} = \text{step/min}$$

Edward must perform 29 stepping cycles per minute to achieve 45 ml O_2/kg/min. To help the subject maintain a consistent pace, a metronome will be set to click at 116 clicks per minute (29 × 4 foot placements = 116 clicks/min).

As you progress through the practice problems for this chapter, it may be helpful to check your estimation answers against Table 11.1.

Chapter 11 Practice Problems

1. Given the following information, determine the total $\dot{V}O_2$.

	Horiz $\dot{V}O_2$ (ml O_2/kg/min)	Vert $\dot{V}O_2$ (ml O_2/kg/min)
(a)	8	12
(b)	12	30

2. Using Table 11.1, determine relative $\dot{V}O_2$ and METs for the following.

	Step height	Stepping rate
(a)	0.254 m	24 step/min
(b)	14 in	128 metronome clicks/min
(c)	0.457 m	36 step/min

3. Determine horizontal $\dot{V}O_2$ when given the following.
   (a) 20 step/min
   (b) 30 step/min

4. Determine vertical $\dot{V}O_2$ component when given the following.
   (a) 20 step/min, .52 m/step
   (b) 25 step/min, .50 m/step

5. Using the entire stepping equation, determine total $\dot{V}O_2$.

	Step height	Step/min
(a)	0.203 m	30
(b)	0.356 m	24

6. Use the following information to solve for height of step (m/step).

$$\text{Vert } \dot{V}O_2 = ?\ \frac{\text{m}}{\text{step}} \times \frac{\text{step}}{\text{min}} \times \frac{2.4 \text{ ml } O_2/\text{kg/min}}{\text{m/min}}$$

	Vert $\dot{V}O_2$ (ml O_2/kg/min)	Step/min
(a)	45	30
(b)	32	35

7. Using the entire bench stepping equation, solve for total $\dot{V}O_2$. After you perform the math, Table 11.1 can be used to check your answers. When using Table 11.1 you may have to interpolate your values between the values in the table.

	m/step	Step/min
(a)	.45	28
(b)	.40	32

8. Solve for step/min using the entire bench step equation.

	Total $\dot{V}O_2$ (ml O_2/kg/min)	Bench height as m/step
(a)	38.38	.254
(b)	43.00	.380

9. Complete the following stepping equation chart.

Use $\frac{39.37 \text{ in}}{1 \text{ m}}$ as the conversion factor.

$$\text{Horiz } \dot{V}O_2 = \frac{\text{step}}{\text{min}} \times \frac{.35 \text{ ml } O_2/\text{kg}/\text{min}}{\text{step}/\text{min}}$$

$$\text{Vert } \dot{V}O_2 = \frac{\text{m}}{\text{step}} \times \frac{\text{step}}{\text{min}} \times \frac{2.4 \text{ ml } O_2/\text{kg}/\text{min}}{\text{m}/\text{min}}$$

Stepping equation chart. The question mark represents the missing value.

	(ml O_2/kg/min)				
	Horiz $\dot{V}O_2$	**Vert $\dot{V}O_2$**	**Total $\dot{V}O_2$**	**Step/min**	**m/step**
(a)	8.4	?	34.9	?	.46 (18 in)
(b)	?	33.60	43.4	28	? (19.69 in)
(c)	10.5	?	32.1	?	.30 (12 in)
(d)	?	?	?	32	.30

10. Determine metronome settings (clicks/min) for each of the following step cycles/min

	Step cycles/min	Metronome setting
(a)	22	?
(b)	26	?
(c)	28	?
(d)	38	?

11. Each $\dot{V}O_2$ answer from any of the ACSM equations represents an estimation. With this in mind, estimate total $\dot{V}O_2$ based upon height of steps and rate of stepping. Use Table 11.1 for each of the following. Round off the $\dot{V}O_2$ values to the nearest whole number.

Height of step	Rate of stepping
(a) 12 in	24 steps/min
(b) .457 m	144 clicks/min (metronome)
(c) .305 m	28 steps/min
(d) 8 in	112 clicks/min

12. Carol, who weighs 127.6 lb, exercises at a rate of 30 steps/min on a 10-in bench. She does this for 15 min each workout. Solve for

(a) Total relative $\dot{V}O_2$

(b) Total absolute $\dot{V}O_2$

(c) kcal/min

(d) kcal for 15 min

(e) kcal for 5 workouts

(f) METs

Chapter 11 Answers to Practice Problems

1. Answers are in the units ml O_2/kg/min.

   (a) 20

   (b) 42

2.

	$\dot{V}O_2$ (ml O_2/kg/min)	METs
(a)	23.03	6.58
(b)	38.54	11.01
(c)	52.08	14.88

3. (a) 7 ml O_2/kg/min

   (b) 10.5 ml O_2/kg/min

4. (a) $\frac{.52\ \cancel{m}}{\cancel{step}} \times \frac{20\ \cancel{step}}{\cancel{min}} \times \frac{2.4\ ml\ O_2/kg/\cancel{min}}{\cancel{m}/min} = \frac{24.96\ ml\ O_2/kg}{min}$

   (b) 30 ml O_2/kg/min

5. (a) 25.1160 ml O_2/kg/min

   (b) 28.9056 ml O_2/kg/min

6. Height of step, vert $\dot{V}O_2$

   (a) .625 m/step (math check: 45/72 = .625)

   (b) .38 m/step

7. Total $\dot{V}O_2$ (ml O_2/kg/min)

   (a) 40.04

   (b) 41.92

8. Step/min

   (a) 40 (math check: $\frac{\text{total } \dot{V}O_2}{.9596}$, (0.254 × 2.4) + 0.35 = .9596)

   (b) 34.07

9. Bench step chart

	Horiz $\dot{V}O_2$	Vert $\dot{V}O_2$	Total $\dot{V}O_2$	Step/min	m/step
(a)	8.4	26.50	34.9	24	.46 (18 in)
(b)	9.8	33.60	43.4	28	.50 (19.69 in)
(c)	10.5	21.60	32.1	30	.30 (12 in)
(d)	11.2	23.04	34.24	30	.30

10. Metronome setting (clicks/min)

    (a) 22 steps/min = 88 clicks/min

    (b) 26 = 104

    (c) 28 = 112

    (d) 38 = 152

11. Total $\dot{V}O_2$ (ml O_2/kg/min) from Table 11.1
    (a) 26
    (b) 52
    (c) 30
    (d) 23
12. Carol's stepping workouts
    (a) Total relative $\dot{V}O_2$ = 28.788 ml O_2/kg/min (Don't round off yet.)
    (b) Total absolute $\dot{V}O_2$ = 1,669.704 ml O_2/min (Don't round off yet.)
    (c) 8.34852 kcal/min (Don't round off yet.)
    (d) 125.2278 kcal expended in 15 min (Don't round off yet.)
    (e) 626.139 kcal expended in 5 workouts, rounded off to 626 kcal
    (f) 8.23 METS

12 Submaximal Exercise Testing and Related Math

Major Concepts

Plotting heart rate-workload points to predict $\dot{V}O_2max$

Submaximal testing with the cycle, treadmill, and bench step to predict $\dot{V}O_2max$

Three equations for estimating $\dot{V}O_2max$

In chapter 1 we considered direct methods of measuring $\dot{V}O_2max$, and in chapters 7, 8, and 9 the methods of estimating $\dot{V}O_2$ using walking and running field testing. In this chapter our focus is on the math and physiology concepts related to *submaximal* exercise testing using the treadmill, cycle, and stepping ergometers for predicting and estimating $\dot{V}O_2max$.

The term GXT, when referred to in the literature, most often is associated with maximal effort testing. However, GXT can apply to submaximal testing as well; any of the maximal GXT protocols can be used as a submaximal exercise test. Submaximal exercise tests can be used for predicting $\dot{V}O_2max$ by taking advantage of the linear relationship between heart rate response and workload $\dot{V}O_2$ values. This linear relationship, as illustrated in Figure 12.1, is most reproducible at low to moderate workloads, between the heart rate values of about 110 and 160 bt/min. At more intense workloads that are at or above the anaerobic threshold, the HR-workload relationship becomes nonlinear.

The HR-workload-$\dot{V}O_2$ linear relationship applies mainly to submaximal workloads approaching the lactate-anaerobic threshold. Each subject may demonstrate slightly different HR-workload points and a slightly different slope angle, but most healthy subjects will show a definite linear relationship between HR, $\dot{V}O_2$ consumption, and workload.

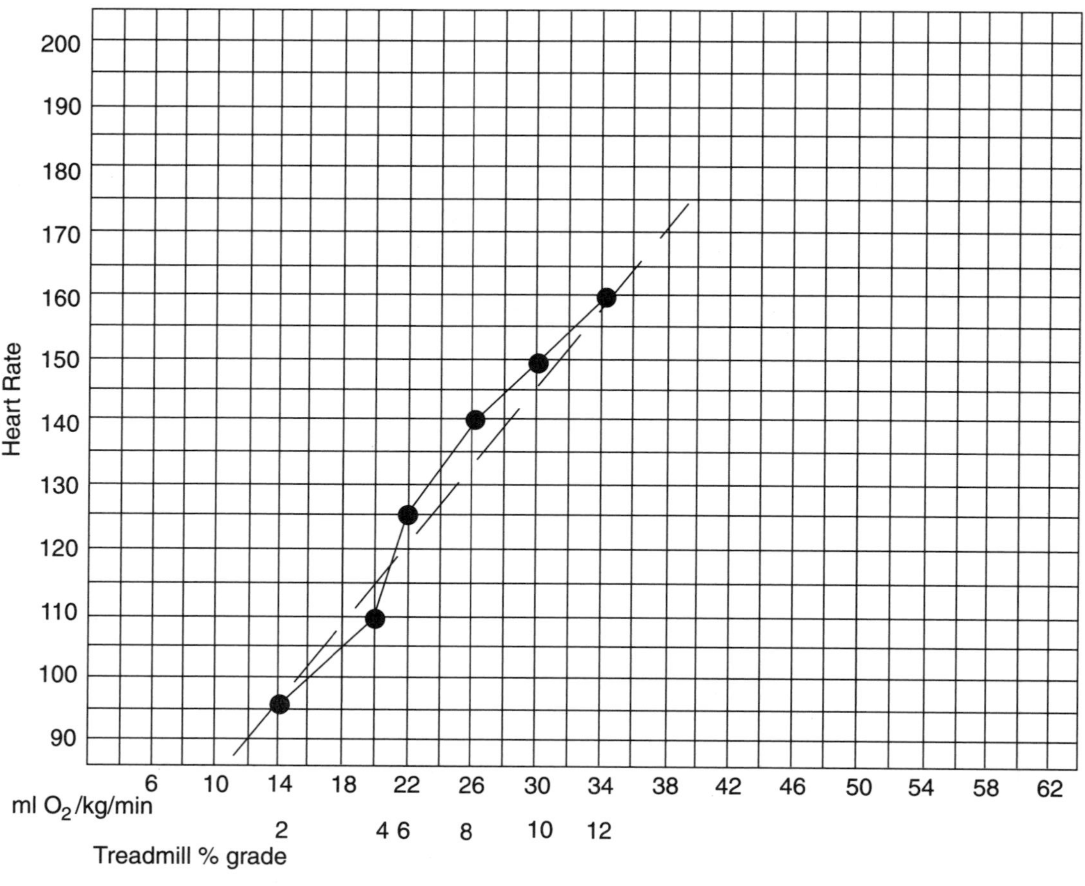

Figure 12.1 An illustration of the linear relationship between heart rate and progressive workload–$\dot{V}O_2$ values. The dashed line is extrapolated through the solid line of actual HR–$\dot{V}O_2$ values from a treadmill submaximal test.

Plotting HR-Workload Points Onto a Graph (Grid) System

After a submaximal test using any of the GXT protocols has been completed, HR and $\dot{V}O_2$ or workload combinations are plotted onto a graph. A suggested approach is to plot the last two HR-workload combinations obtained. The last HR-workload combination should be as near as possible to 85% of 220 − age (Karvonen heart rate reserve method). (Follow Figure 12.2 throughout this discussion.)

When the last two plots are recorded onto the graph, draw a straight line connecting the plots. For best results the first plotted point must be above the HR of 110 bt/min. The line between the last two plots is then extended up to the horizontal line that represents the subject's maximal HR (220 − age).

From the intersection of the two lines, drop another line straight down to the x-axis (baseline) marked with workloads. The workload or $\dot{V}O_2$ at the bottom of the vertical line represents the subject's estimated (predicted) $\dot{V}O_2$max. Table 12.1 will help you convert cycle workloads on the horizontal (bottom) axis to $\dot{V}O_2$ values and METs based upon a subject's body weight and a pedaling speed of 50 rev/min.

In the treadmill/bench stepping graph, the $\dot{V}O_2$ values (ml O_2/kg/min) are listed along the baseline. Appendix D provides a table of $\dot{V}O_2$ values that are already calculated based upon treadmill speed and elevation. With the cycle ergometer

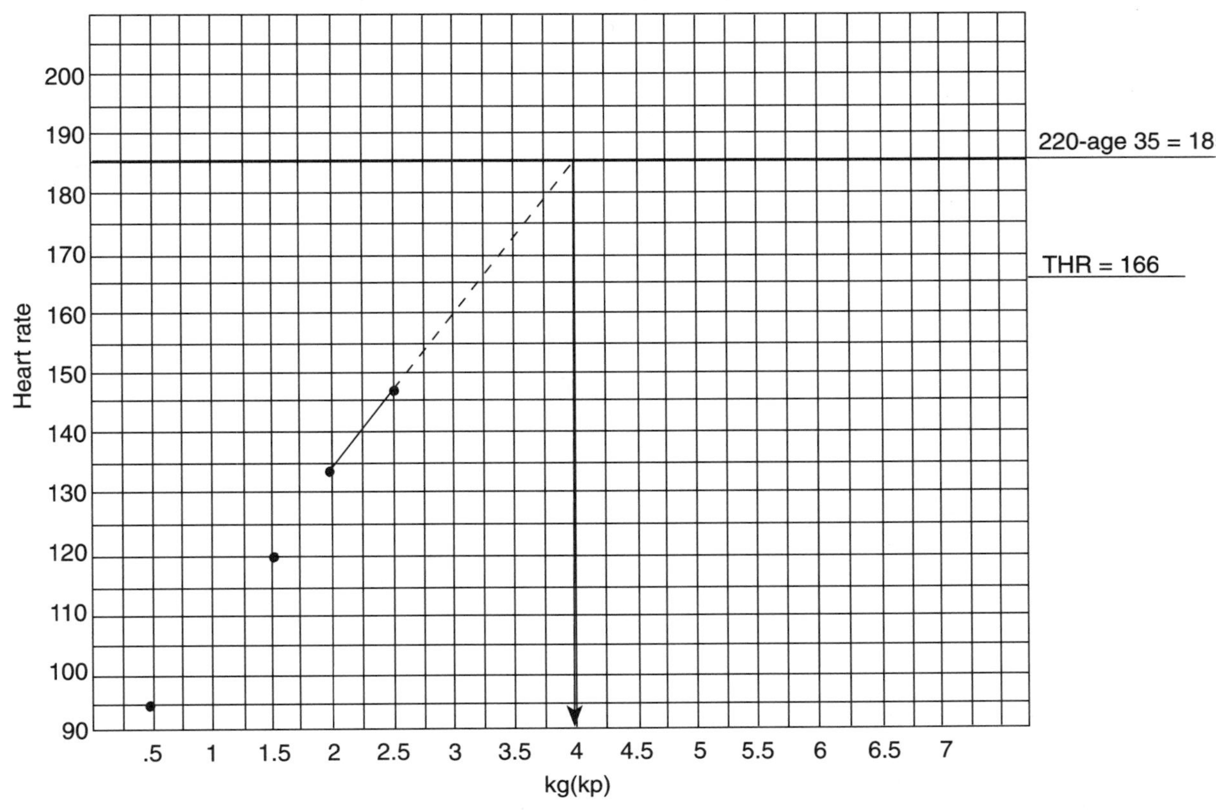

Figure 12.2 Estimating $\dot{V}O_2$max by graphing. See Table 12.4 for $\dot{V}O_2$ values that correspond to subject's body weight.

graph, the horizontal axis (baseline) maximal workload (kgm/min) must be entered into the cycle equation (chapter 10) to arrive at the $\dot{V}O_2$max. Let's do an example problem to see how this works.

Example 12A

Graph to estimate $\dot{V}O_2$max from cycle test. Ken is 35 years old, weighs 80 kg, and has a resting HR of 60 bt/min. He has just completed a submaximal cycle test using the YMCA branching protocol outlined in Table 12.4. (The YMCA branching protocols are shown in Tables 12.2, 12.3, and 12.4 on pp. 162, 163). The results of Ken's test follow.

Ken's Test Results

Stage	Workload	Heart rate (bt/min)	Blood pressure
1st	150 kgm/min 0.5 kp	94	120/70
2nd	450 kgm/min 1.5 kp	120	130/70
3rd	600 kgm/min 2.0 kp	134	142/66
4th	750 kgm/min 2.5 kp	146	170/60

Table 12.1 Table to Estimate (Predict) $\dot{V}O_2max$ From Submaximal (Leg) Cycle Workloads (Pedaling Speed = 50 rev/min)

kg(kp) **kgm/min**	**1** **300**	**1.5**	**2** **600**	**2.5**	**3** **900**	**3.5**	**4** **1,200**	**4.5**	**5** **1,500**	**5.5**	**6** **1,800**	**6.5**	**7** **2,100**
O_2 constant in cycle equation ml O_2/kgm	2.0	2.0	2.0	2.0	2.0	2.0	2.09	2.14	2.16	2.17	2.19	2.22	2.24
wt = 60 kg (132 lb)													
ml O_2/min	810		1,410		2,010		2,718		3,450		4,152		4,914
ml O_2/kg/min	13.5		23.5		33.5		45.3		57.5		69.2		81.9
METs	3.8		6.7		9.6		12.9		16.4		19.8		23.4
wt = 70 kg (154 lb)													
ml O_2/min	845		1,445		2,045		2,753		3,485		4,187		4,949
ml O_2/kg/min	12		20.6		29.2		39.3		49.8		59.8		70.7
METs	3.4		5.9		8.3		11.2		14.2		17.1		20.2
wt = 80 kg (176 lb)													
ml O_2/min	880		1,480		2,080		2,788		3,520		4,222		4,984
ml O_2/kg/min	11		18.5		26		34.9		44		52.8		62.3
METs	3.1		5.3		7.4		10		12.6		15.1		17.8
wt = 86 kg (189.2 lb)													
L O_2/min	.901	1.2	1.5	1.8	2.1	2.4	2.8	3.2	3.5	3.8	4.2	4.6	5.0
ml O_2/min	901	1,201	1,501	1,801	2,101	2,401	2,809	3,190	3,541	3,882	4,243	4,630	5,005
ml O_2/kg/min	10.5	14.0	17.4	20.9	24.4	28.0	32.7	37.1	41.2	45.1	49.3	53.8	58.2
METs	3.0	4.0	5.0	6.0	7.0	8.0	9.3	10.6	11.8	12.9	14.1	15.4	16.6

Step 1: Find the THR using the Karvonen formula.
220 − 35 = 185
185 − 60 bt/min (RHR) = 125 bt/min
125 bt/min × .85 = 106 bt/min
106 bt/min + 60 bt/min = 166 bt/min THR

The test was stopped at a heart rate of 146 bt/min.

Step 2: Plot the results.
Figure 12.2 shows how Ken's HR-workload combinations are plotted. The two HR-workload plots, 134 bt/min (2 kp) and 146 bt/min (2.5 kp), are connected by a solid straight line. This line is extended (dashed line) up to the horizontal HRmax line of 185 bt/min (220 − age 35 = 185). At this intersection of lines a vertical line is dropped down to a point on the baseline corresponding to a predicted maximal workload of 4.0 kp.

Step 3: Estimate $\dot{V}O_2max$.
By checking Table 12.1 you'll find that Ken's $\dot{V}O_2max$ is 34.9 ml O_2/kg/min or 10 METs. Table 12.1 was calculated using the cycle equation from chapter 10.

Submaximal Exercise Test Examples

What follows is a set of example problems illustrating methods of submaximal exercise testing along with brief discussions of the physiological concepts concerning oxygen consumption. There are also examples illustrating *mathematical equations* for predicting $\dot{V}O_2$max.

Treadmill Submaximal Exercise Test

Plotting HR-$\dot{V}O_2$ values onto a graph for a treadmill submaximal exercise test is essentially the same as with cycle ergometer testing. With cycle testing you calculate the $\dot{V}O_2$max from the predicted maximal workload of kgm/min from the horizontal axis by using the cycle equation from chapter 10 or by locating the correct $\dot{V}O_2$ on Table 12.1.

For treadmill testing, each $\dot{V}O_2$ point related to treadmill speed and grade must be calculated from the treadmill walking or running equations (chapters 8 and 9) or the $\dot{V}O_2$ values in the tables in appendix D.

Example 12B

Graph HR-$\dot{V}O_2$ values for a treadmill submaximal GXT. Mr. Smith has completed a submaximal GXT on a treadmill. He is 45 years old and weighs 80 kg. His age-predicted HRmax is 175 bt/min. The stopping point (THR) of this test was 85% of 175 bt/min according to the Karvonen formula (chapter 6); this equals a THR of 158 bt/min. Estimate the $\dot{V}O_2$max.

Test Results

Stage	Time	mph	m/min	Grade (%)	HR (bt/min)	$\dot{V}O_2$ (ml O_2/kg/min)
1	3 min	1.7	45.56	5	114	12.16
2	3 min	1.7	45.56	10	120	16.30
3	3 min	2.5	67.00	12	158	24.67

Step 1: Use the walking equation from chapter 8 or refer to Appendix D to convert stages 2 and 3 into ml O_2/kg/min (For this example this has already been done in the test results table. Check the $\dot{V}O_2$ values in the test table with those in Appendix D.)

Step 2: The HR-$\dot{V}O_2$ combinations from stages 2 and 3 have been plotted onto the graph in Figure 12.3.

Step 3: The solid line between the points of stages 2 and 3 is extended (extrapolated) up to the HRmax line of 175 bt/min using a dashed line.

Step 4: From the intersection of lines, a vertical line is drawn down to the baseline to meet the $\dot{V}O_2$max value of 29 ml O_2/kg/min.

Submaximal Bench Step Testing to Predict $\dot{V}O_2$max

There are two basic methods for performing submaximal GXTs using a bench step.

Graphing HR-$\dot{V}O_2$ Values The first method is to graph the HR-$\dot{V}O_2$ values to predict $\dot{V}O_2$max as in treadmill and cycle submaximal testing. With this method,

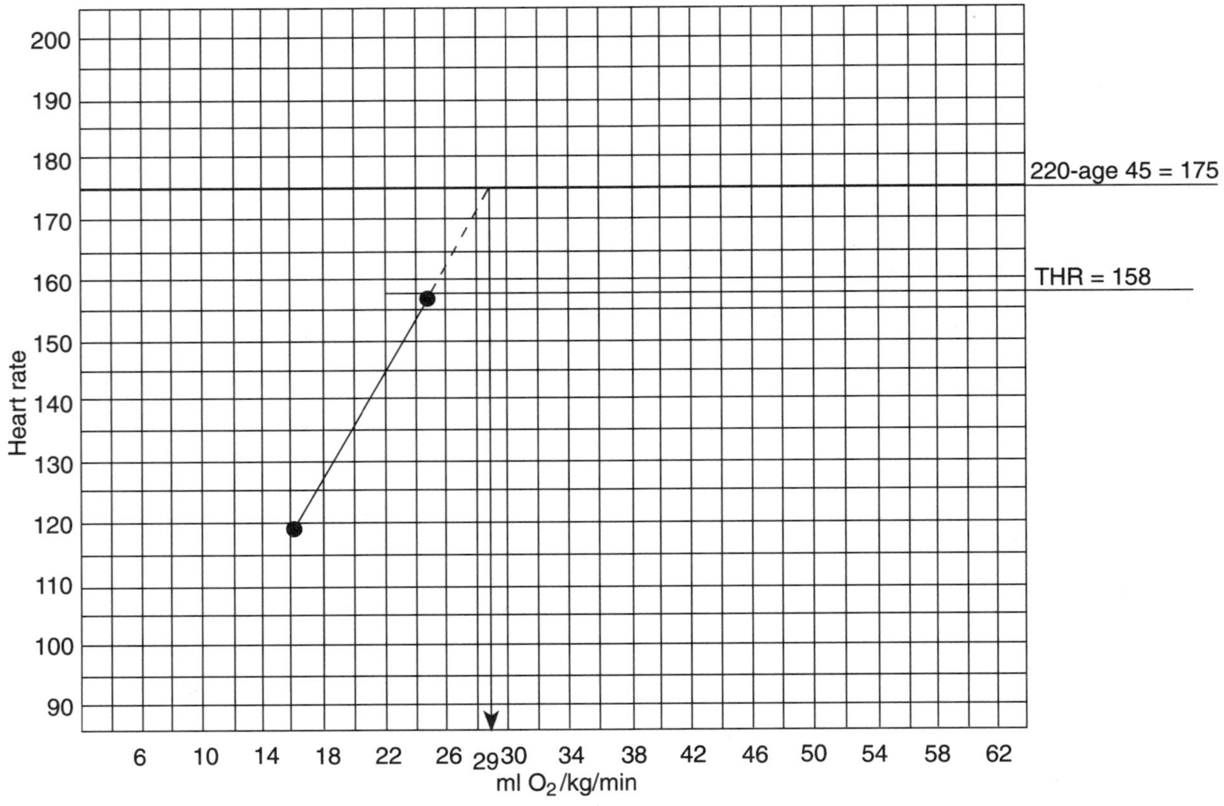

Figure 12.3 Illustration of Example 12B.

step height or cadence, or both, can be increased to provide increasing workloads. The method of plotting HR-$\dot{V}O_2$ combinations is presented in Example 12C.

Example 12C

Plot HR-$\dot{V}O_2$ values on a graph for a bench stepping submaximal test. Karen, age 25, performed a GXT using a 12-in (.30 m) bench with a progressive increase in stepping cadence. Karen's RHR was 60 bt/min. The cadence increased in rate every 2 min.

Test Results

Stage	Metronome cadence/min	HR	$\dot{V}O_2$ (ml O_2/kg/min)
1	20 cycles (80 clicks)	110	21.40
2	25 cycles (100 clicks)	130	26.75
3	30 cycles (120 clicks)	150	32.10
4	35 cycles (140 clicks)	170	37.45

Step 1: Calculate the $\dot{V}O_2$ for each stage using the bench stepping equation from chapter 11.

Step 2: Plot HR-$\dot{V}O_2$ combinations from stages 3 and 4 onto the graph in Figure 12.4.

The predicted $\dot{V}O_2$max for Karen is approximately 43 ml O_2/kg/min (12.3 METs).

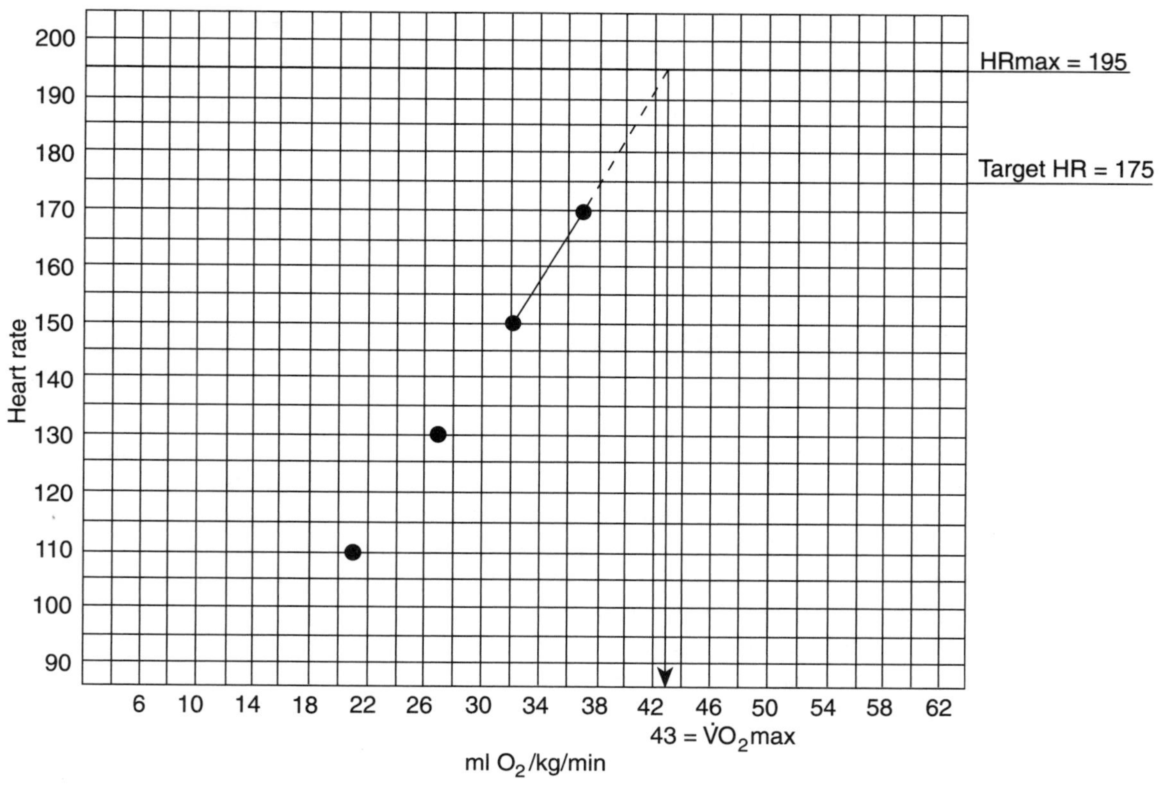

Figure 12.4 Illustration of Example 12C.

Using recovery heart rate to estimate $\dot{V}O_2$max The second method of performing a submaximal step test to estimate $\dot{V}O_2$max is based upon recovery heart rate (McArdle, Katch, Pechar, Jacobson, & Ruck, 1972), as you will see in Example 12D. After the subject steps for 3 min, the HR is recorded for 15 sec and multiplied by 4 to yield a 1-min HR. As you can see by looking at the equations of McArdle et al. below, the male equation has a much larger constant number (111.33), related to a male's greater muscle mass. The constant in the female equation is 65.81.

$$\text{Predicted } \dot{V}O_2\text{max (males)} = 111.33 - (0.42 \times \text{1-min HR})$$
$$\text{Predicted } \dot{V}O_2\text{max (females)} = 65.81 - (0.1847 \times \text{1-min HR})$$

To predict an estimation of $\dot{V}O_2$max, the 1-min recovery HR is entered into the appropriate equation.

The female $\dot{V}O_2$ prediction equation is used in example 12D.

Example 12D

Predict $\dot{V}$O2max using the 3-min submaximal bench step test. Janet performed the 3-min step test. After she finished, her radial pulse was 32 beats for 15 sec. Predict her $\dot{V}O_2$max.

Step 1: Multiply Janet's 15-sec pulse by 4 to find bt/min.

$$32 \times 4 = 128 \text{ bt/min}$$

Step 2: Enter the HR into the equation of McArdle et al. for females to estimate $\dot{V}O_2max$, as follows.

$$\dot{V}O_2max\text{ (female)} = 65.81 - (0.1847 \times \text{1-min HR of 128 bt/min})$$
$$\dot{V}O_2max\text{ (female)} = 65.81 - 23.64$$
$$\dot{V}O_2max\text{ (female)} = 42.17\text{ ml } O_2/\text{kg/min}$$

Compare this $\dot{V}O_2max$ with the results in example 12C.

Three Equations for Predicting $\dot{V}O_2max$ From Submaximal Exercise Testing

A submaximal exercise test is used to determine the slope angle of the linear relationship between HR and workload and $\dot{V}O_2$, as was demonstrated in the previous section by drawing the slope of a line onto a graph. A mathematical equation can be used to calculate a subject's HR-workload slope and predict $\dot{V}O_2max$. You can memorize one of the following equations and use it during exercise physiology exams to estimate $\dot{V}O_2max$ when a graphing system is not available.

These three equations are easy to remember and can be used with cycle and treadmill submaximal testing:

- Single HR-$\dot{V}O_2$ equation (Mahar, 1985)
- Double HR-$\dot{V}O_2$ equation (Shephard 1970, 1972)
- THR-$\dot{V}O_2$ equation (Pollock, Wilmore, & Fox, 1978)

When Mahar (1985) compared the single HR-$\dot{V}O_2$ equation with the double HR-$\dot{V}O_2$ equation (Shephard, 1970), he found that they provided similar answers when estimating $\dot{V}O_2max$.

Single HR-$\dot{V}O_2$ Equation

This equation (Mahar, 1985) considers gender and age and is most accurate with treadmill and cycle submaximal testing. HRmax is calculated using a subject's age.

$$\text{Men:}\quad \text{Estimated } \dot{V}O_2max = (\text{final } \dot{V}O_2) \times \left(\frac{\text{HRmax} - 61}{\text{final HR} - 61}\right)$$

$$\text{Women: Estimated } \dot{V}O_2max = (\text{final } \dot{V}O_2) \times \left(\frac{\text{HRmax} - 72}{\text{final HR} - 72}\right)$$

where final $\dot{V}O_2$ is the highest $\dot{V}O_2$ during the final workload of the submaximal test, HRmax is 220 minus age, and final HR is the heart rate that corresponds to the final $\dot{V}O_2$. The numbers 61 and 72 represent the average RHRs (bt/min) of the men and women, respectively, in Mahar's study. Example 12E provides an illustration of Mahar's prediction equation.

Example 12E

Use the single HR-$\dot{V}O_2$ equation to predict $\dot{V}O_2max$. Doug, age 35, weighs 80 kg and has a RHR of 60 bpm. He completed a submaximal cycle test while pedaling at a speed of 50 rev/min. His test was stopped at a final workload of 3 kp (900 kgm/min). At this point, Doug's HR was 166 bt/min. Use the given information to calculate an estimation of $\dot{V}O_2max$.

Step 1: Find HRmax.

$$\text{HRmax} = 220 - \text{age } 35 = 185 \text{ bt/min}$$

Step 2: Insert information into the male equation.

$$\text{Est. } \dot{V}O_2\text{max} = (\text{final } \dot{V}O_2) \times \left(\frac{\text{HRmax} - 61 \text{ bt/min}}{\text{final HR} - 61 \text{ bt/min}}\right)$$

$$\text{Est. } \dot{V}O_2\text{max} = (2{,}080 \text{ ml } O_2/\text{min}) \times \left(\frac{185 \text{ bt/min} - 61 \text{ bt/min}}{166 \text{ bt/min} - 61 \text{ bt/min}}\right)$$

$$\text{Est. } \dot{V}O_2\text{max} = 2{,}080 \text{ ml } O_2/\text{min} \times 1.1809523 \text{ (Do not round off.)}$$

$$\text{Est. } \dot{V}O_2\text{max} = 2{,}456.38 \text{ ml } O_2/\text{min, at } 80 \text{ kg} = 30.7 \text{ ml } O_2/\text{kg/min}$$

Step 3: From Table 12.1 you can see that the value 30.7 ml O_2/kg/min falls about halfway between the values 26 and 34.9 ml O_2/kg/min. The value 30.7 ml O_2/kg/min is about 8.77 METs.

The final workload for Doug was 3 kp. His predicted maximal workload is at 3.5 kp (30.7 ml O_2/kg/min). His predicted maximal workload is slightly higher than his final workload, by .5 kp. If you go back and calculate Doug's THR using the Karvonen formula, you will find that it is very near the heart rate of 166 that was the stopping point of his test. Remember, these are methods for arriving at an estimated $\dot{V}O_2$max.

Double HR-$\dot{V}O_2$ Equation

The double HR-$\dot{V}O_2$ equation (Shephard, 1970, 1972) uses two sequential HR-$\dot{V}O_2$ values and can be used with cycle as well as treadmill submaximal testing. For most accurate estimation of $\dot{V}O_2$max, the two $\dot{V}O_2$ values must match with two HR values between the heart rates of 115 and 150 bt/min. This calculation considers age but no gender, so there is only one equation.

$$\dot{V}O_2\text{max} = (\text{2nd } \dot{V}O_2) + \left[\left(\frac{\text{2nd } \dot{V}O_2 - \text{1st } \dot{V}O_2}{\text{2nd HR} - \text{1st HR}}\right) \times (\text{HRmax} - \text{2nd HR})\right]$$

where 2nd $\dot{V}O_2$ is the $\dot{V}O_2$ value from the second HR-$\dot{V}O_2$ combination; 1st $\dot{V}O_2$ is the $\dot{V}O_2$ value from the first HR-$\dot{V}O_2$ combination ($\dot{V}O_2$ values can be in the units ml O_2/kg/min, ml O_2/min, or METs.); 2nd HR is the HR from the second HR-$\dot{V}O_2$ combination; and 1st HR is the HR from the first HR-$\dot{V}O_2$ combination.

Example 12F

Predict $\dot{V}O_2$max using the double HR-$\dot{V}O_2$ equation. Susan (age 30) has completed a GXT on a treadmill. Treadmill speed was at a constant 3.3 mph. The results of the test follow.

Test Results

Stage	Grade (%)	$\dot{V}O_2$ (ml O_2/kg/min)	HR (bt/min)
1	2	Not needed	90
2	4	Not needed	102
3	6	Not needed	108
4	8	Not needed	112
5	10	Not needed	124
6	12	Not needed	132
7	14	34.63 (1st $\dot{V}O_2$)	140 (1st HR)
8	16	37.81 (2nd $\dot{V}O_2$)	150 (2nd HR)

$\dot{V}O_2$ for stages 7 and 8 can be calculated on the basis of speed and grade using the walking equation, chapter 8, or using appendix D. Stage 7 represents the 1st $\dot{V}O_2$ and the 1st HR. Stage 8 represents the 2nd $\dot{V}O_2$ and the 2nd HR.

Step 1: Find Susan's HRmax

$$\text{HRmax} = 220 - \text{age } 30 = 190 \text{ bt/min.}$$

Step 2: Enter the correct information into the double HR-$\dot{V}O_2$ equation.

$$\dot{V}O_2\text{max} = (\text{2nd } \dot{V}O_2) + \left[\left(\frac{\text{2nd } \dot{V}O_2 - \text{1st } \dot{V}O_2}{\text{2nd HR} - \text{1st HR}}\right) \times (\text{HRmax} - \text{2nd HR})\right]$$

$$\dot{V}O_2\text{max} = (37.81 \text{ ml } O_2/\text{kg/min}) + \left[\left(\frac{37.81 \text{ ml } O_2/\text{kg/min} - 34.63 \text{ ml } O_2/\text{kg/min}}{150 \text{ bt/min} - 140 \text{ bt/min}}\right) \times (190 \text{ bt/min} - 150 \text{ bt/min})\right]$$

$$\dot{V}O_2\text{max} = (37.81 \text{ ml } O_2/\text{kg/min}) + \left(\frac{.318 \text{ ml } O_2/\text{kg/min}}{\text{bt/min}} \times 40 \text{ bt/min}\right)$$

$$\dot{V}O_2\text{max} = 50.53 \text{ ml } O_2/\text{kg/min or } 14.44 \text{ METs}$$

THR-$\dot{V}O_2$ Equation

The THR-$\dot{V}O_2$ equation (Pollock et al., 1978) requires that the subject reach the THR before the test is stopped. THR is 85% of HRmax using the Karvonen formula. In this respect it differs from the single and double HR-$\dot{V}O_2$ equations illustrated in Examples 12E and 12F. The Pollock THR-$\dot{V}O_2$ equation considers age and final $\dot{V}O_2$, but not gender. This equation, which is applicable with cycle and treadmill submaximal testing, is:

$$\dot{V}O_2\text{max} = \text{final } \dot{V}O_2 \times 1.174$$

where final $\dot{V}O_2$ is the $\dot{V}O_2$ that occurs at the time the subject reaches the THR and 1.174 is a constant that represents the average linear slope line of heart rate and $\dot{V}O_2$ combinations from the group of subjects studied by Pollock et al.

Example 12G illustrates the use of the THR-$\dot{V}O_2$ equation.

Example 12G

Predict $\dot{V}O_2$max using the THR-$\dot{V}O_2$ equation. William, age 45, weighs 70 kg and has a RHR of 50 bt/min. He performed a submaximal GXT on a cycle ergometer.

The branching YMCA protocol (Table 12.2) for males was used for this test. The workload of 1,200 kgm/min brought William's HR up to a steady-state rate of 156 bt/min (his THR), which was the cue to stop this submaximal test.

Step 1: From Table 12.1, find the final $\dot{V}O_2$ that corresponds to the workload Ken reached.

Table 12.1 shows that a workload of 1,200 kgm/min (4 kp) for a 70-kg subject is a $\dot{V}O_2$ of 39.3 ml O_2/kg/min or 11.2 METs.

Step 2: Enter the appropriate information into the equation.

$$\dot{V}O_2\text{max} = \text{final } \dot{V}O_2 \times 1.174$$
$$\dot{V}O_2\text{max} = 39.3 \text{ ml } O_2/\text{kg/min} \times 1.174$$
$$\dot{V}O_2\text{max} = 46.14 \text{ ml } O_2/\text{kg/min}$$

You can see how Pollock et al. (1978) arrived at the constant of 1.174. Look at step 2 in Example 12E, the Mahar (1985) single HR-$\dot{V}O_2$ equation. The number 1.174 from the equation of Pollock et al. is very close to 1.180 in the Mahar equation.

Figures 12.5 and 12.6 are blank graphs (grids) to be used for predicting $\dot{V}O_2$max when performing submaximal exercise testing with a cycle or treadmill and bench step ergometers.

Figure 12.5 is the cycle ergometer graph. Use this graph to plot HR-workload combinations when performing submaximal testing using a cycle ergometer. The baseline of Figure 12.5 is used in conjunction with Table 12.1 for determination of $\dot{V}O_2$ based upon a subject's body weight and pedaling resistance. Table 12.1 was prepared using the cycle equation from chapter 10.

Note that when performing submaximal testing using an arm ergometer, you must perform your own math calculations to arrive at $\dot{V}O_2$ and MET values. Use the arm ergometer equation from chapter 10.

Figure 12.6 is the treadmill ergometer graph. This graph can be used to plot HR-$\dot{V}O_2$ combinations when performing treadmill and stepping submaximal testing. See appendix D for a table of $\dot{V}O_2$ values related to treadmill elevation and speed.

To arrive at $\dot{V}O_2$ values during a stepping test, as in example 12C, you must calculate your own $\dot{V}O_2$ values based upon step height and rate of stepping using the stepping equation from chapter 11.

You are welcome to make copies of these blank graphs to be used when performing the practice problems at the end of this chapter or when conducting submaximal testing at your own facility.

Summary

Submaximal exercise testing is used to predict an estimation of maximal aerobic capacity on the basis of a single HR-$\dot{V}O_2$/workload combination or a series of HR-$\dot{V}O_2$ combinations during submaximal exercise testing. This method takes advantage of the linear relationship between HR response and workload values.

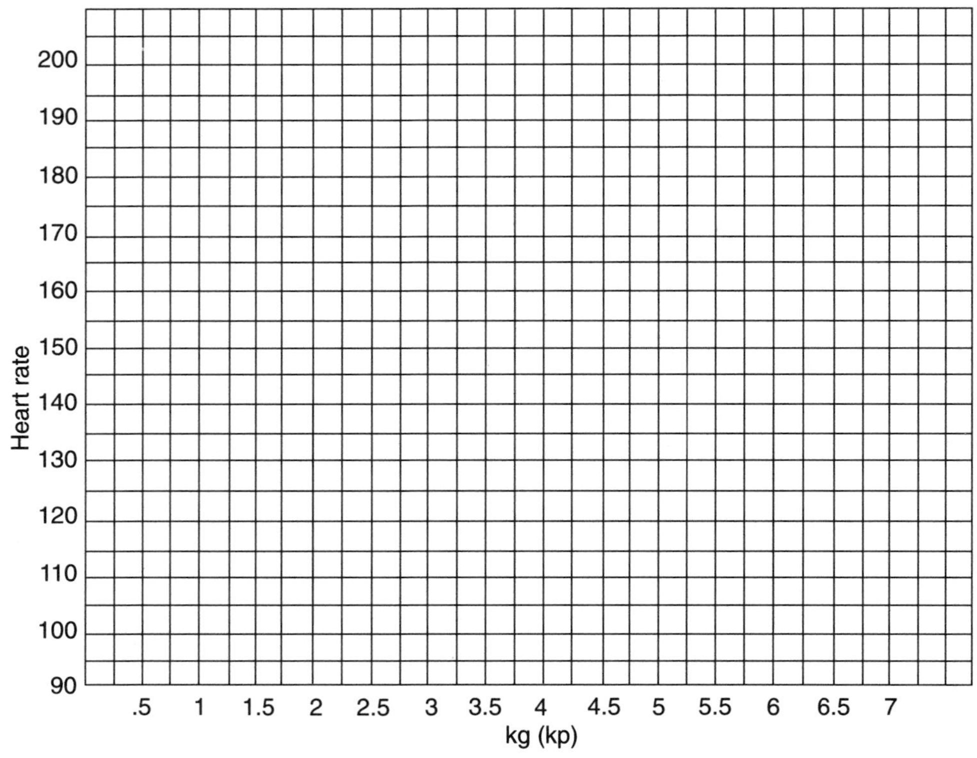

Figure 12.5 Plotting HR–workload points from submaximal cycle testing.

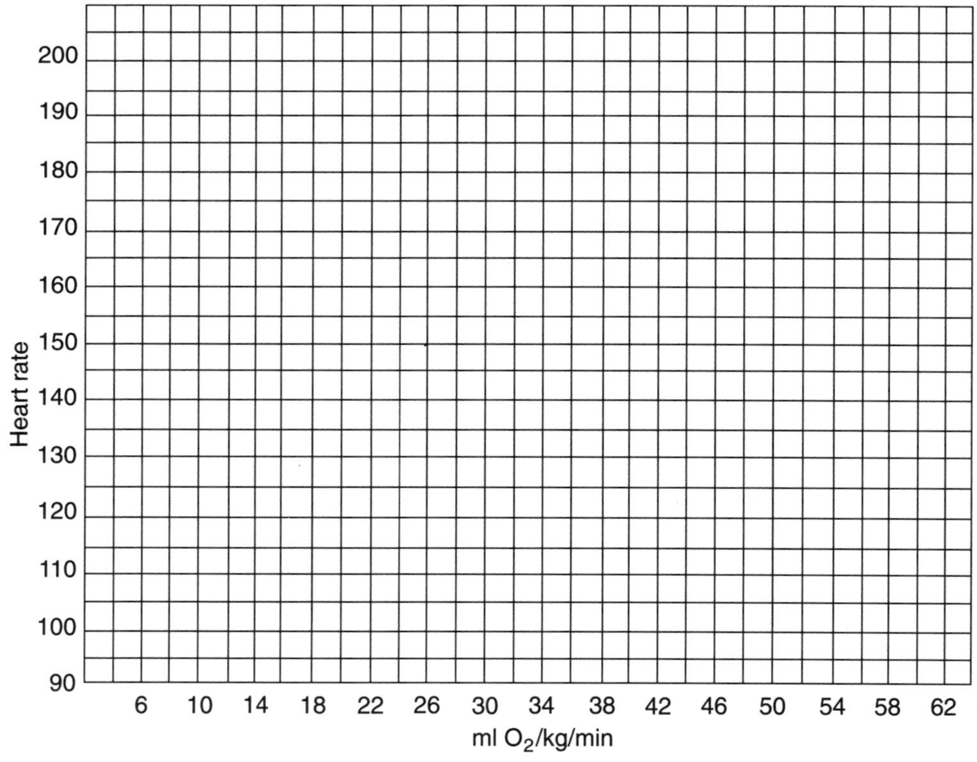

Figure 12.6 Plotting $\dot{V}O_2$max from submaximal treadmill and bench step testing.

Chapter 12 Practice Problems

The question mark in some of these problems indicates missing piece(s) of information. You are to find the missing pieces or missing numbers.

1. Use Table 12.1 to complete the following chart.

kp	kgm/min	wt (kg)	ml O_2/min	ml O_2/kg/min	METs
1	300	60	?	?	3.8
2	600	?	?	18.5	5.3
3.5	?	86	2,401	?	?

2. Jeff, who weighs 80 kg, performed a submaximal cycle test. His predicted maximal workload was 5 kp (1,500 kgm/min). What is his estimated $\dot{V}O_2max$? Use Table 12.1 to find the answer.

3. Susan performed a submaximal cycle ergometer test. Her weight is 64 kg. Her predicted maximal workload was 3 kp (900 kgm/min). Use the cycle equation to determine her estimated $\dot{V}O_2max$.

4. For this question refer to Table 12.3, the YMCA branching cycle protocol for females or unfit males.

   Alexis, 32 years old, is performing a submaximal cycle test using the YMCA branching protocol for females. At the end of the 1st workload Alexis's heart rate was greater than 103. At the end of her 2nd workload her heart rate is at a steady state of 136 bt/min.

   (a) What is her next workload in kgm/min and kp?

   (b) What is her correct pedaling speed for this YMCA protocol?

   (c) What is her age-predicted HRmax?

5. David performed a submaximal cycle test. Use the blank cycle graph (Figure 12.5) to plot his submaximal cycle test workloads and HRs. David's weight = 86 kg and his age = 40. The YMCA protocol for males and females of average fitness level (Table 12.4) was used for this test. Plot stages 3 and 4 and predict David's $\dot{V}O_2max$.

Test Results

Stage	HR	Workload
1	112	0.5 kp (150 kgm/min)
2	124	1.0 kp (300 kgm/min)
3	135	1.5 kp (450 kgm/min)
4	145	2.0 kp (600 kgm/min)

   Plug David's predicted maximal workload (horizontal base line) into the cycle equation to determine estimated $\dot{V}O_2max$ in ml O_2/min, absolute.

Table 12.2 The Y's Way to Physical Fitness Submaximal Exercise Testing Branching Protocol for Males or for Very Fit Females

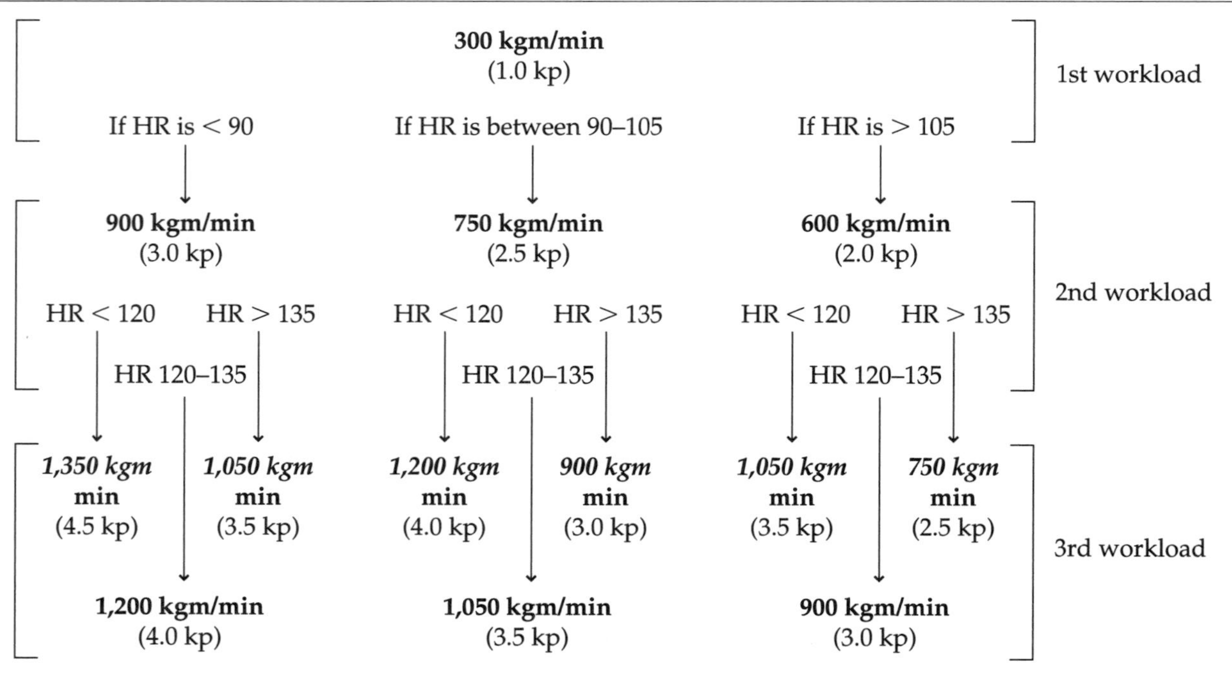

6. Use Appendix D to find the $\dot{V}O_2$ (ml O_2/kg/min, relative) for the following treadmill walking percent grades and speeds.

% Grade	Speed	$\dot{V}O_2$ (ml O_2/kg/min)
2	3.0 mph	?
4	3.4 mph	?
0 (flat)	187.60 m/min	?

7. Lisa, age 45, has just completed a submaximal GXT using the Bruce treadmill protocol (Table 8.2). Use the treadmill grid in Figure 12.6 to plot the HR-$\dot{V}O_2$ combinations and predict her $\dot{V}O_2$max. Plot stages 2 and 3. HRmax = 220 − age 45 = 175 bt/min.

Test Results

Stages	% Grade	Speed (mph)	HR	$\dot{V}O_2$
1	10	1.7	105	?
2	12	2.5	125	?
3	14	3.4	150	?

Table 12.3 The Y's Way to Physical Fitness Submaximal Exercise Testing Branching Protocol for Females or Very Unfit Males

1st workload			**150 kgm/min** (0.5 kp)		
	If HR is < 103			If HR is > 103	
2nd workload	**450 kgm/min** (1.5 kp)			**300 kgm/min** (1.0 kp)	
	HR < 138	HR > 138		HR < 123	HR > 123
3rd workload	**250 kgm/min** (2.5 kp)	**600 kgm/min** (2.0 kp)		**600 kgm/min** (2.0 kp)	**450 kgm/min** (1.5 kp)

From *The Y's Way to Physical Fitness: A Guidebook for Instructors* (Rev. ed., p. 91), by L. A. Golding, C. R. Myers, and W. E. Sinning, 1982, Chicago: National Board of the YMCA. Copyright 1982 by the National Board of the YMCA. Reprinted with permission of the YMCA of the USA, 101 N. Wacker Drive, Chicago, IL 60606.

Table 12.4 The Y's Way to Physical Fitness Physical Work Capacity Cycle Test for Male or Female Subjects of Average Level of Fitness

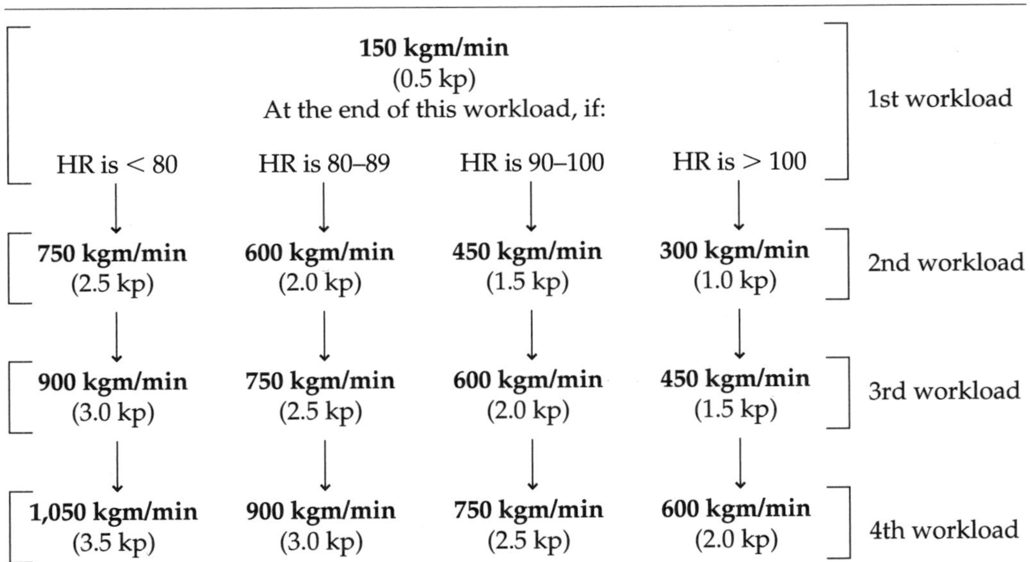

1st workload	**150 kgm/min** (0.5 kp) At the end of this workload, if:			
	HR is < 80	HR is 80–89	HR is 90–100	HR is > 100
2nd workload	**750 kgm/min** (2.5 kp)	**600 kgm/min** (2.0 kp)	**450 kgm/min** (1.5 kp)	**300 kgm/min** (1.0 kp)
3rd workload	**900 kgm/min** (3.0 kp)	**750 kgm/min** (2.5 kp)	**600 kgm/min** (2.0 kp)	**450 kgm/min** (1.5 kp)
4th workload	**1,050 kgm/min** (3.5 kp)	**900 kgm/min** (3.0 kp)	**750 kgm/min** (2.5 kp)	**600 kgm/min** (2.0 kp)

From *The Y's Way to Physical Fitness: A Complete Guide to Fitness Testing and Instruction* (3rd ed., p. 91), by L. A. Golding, C. R. Myers, and W. E. Sinning, 1989, Champaign, IL: Human Kinetics. Copyright 1989 by National Council of Young Men's Christian Associations of the United States of America. Reprinted with permission of the YMCA of the USA, 101 N. Wacker Drive, Chicago, IL 60606.

First, complete the test results table. Determine $\dot{V}O_2$ for each stage. Then plot stages 2 and 3. Extend the line up to the HRmax line. From this point drop a line down to the baseline to find the predicted $\dot{V}O_2$max.

8. Use the treadmill/bench stepping graph (Figure 12.6) to plot the bench stepping HR-$\dot{V}O_2$ combinations.

   Mr. Martens, age 35, completed a submaximal step test. His results are provided in the following table. Bench step height was 12 in (.30 m). Plot stages 2 and 3 to predict $\dot{V}O_2$max.

Test Results

Stage	Cadence (cycles/min)	HR	$\dot{V}O_2$ (ml O_2/kg/min)
1	16	96	?
2	26	126	?
3	36	155	?

Your first step is to calculate $\dot{V}O_2$ for each stage using the stepping equation. Remember, you must add the horizontal $\dot{V}O_2$ to the vertical $\dot{V}O_2$.

$$\text{Horiz } \dot{V}O_2 = \frac{?\text{ step}}{\text{min}} \times \frac{0.35\text{ ml } O_2/\text{kg/min}}{\text{step/min}}$$

$$+\ \text{Vertical } \dot{V}O_2 = \frac{?\text{ m}}{\text{step}} \times \frac{?\text{ step}}{\text{min}} \times \frac{2.4\text{ ml } O_2/\text{kg/min}}{\text{m/min}}$$

$$\text{Total } \dot{V}O_2 = ?\text{ ml } O_2/\text{kg/min}$$

9. Determine the THR (target heart rate) for each of the following subjects. Use the Karvonen formula and complete the table.

Name	Age	Rest HR	% of HRmax	THR
John	25	50	85	?
Karen	40	65	80	?
Cliff	52	70	85	?

10. Holly performed a submaximal 3-min step test using a 16.25-in bench and maintained a stepping rate of 22 step cycles per minute throughout the test. She performed this step test two times over a period of 1 year of fitness training. You have been asked to estimate her $\dot{V}O_2$max for each test using the equation of McArdle et al. (1972).

$$\text{Est. } \dot{V}O_2\text{max (females)} = 65.81 - (0.1847 \times \text{1-min HR})$$

Test Results

Test	15-sec recovery HR	1-min HR	Est. $\dot{V}O_2$max
#1	44	?	?
#2	40	?	?

11. Tom and Ralph both performed the 3-min step test using a 16.25-in bench and stepping at a rate of 24 stepping cycles per minute. Both were able to complete the 3 min of stepping. Use the McArdle equation to estimate their $\dot{V}O_2max$.

$$\text{Est. } \dot{V}O_2max \text{ (males)} = 111.33 - (0.42 \times \text{1-min HR})$$

Name	1-min recovery HR	$\dot{V}O_2max$ (ml O_2/kg/min)
Tom	154 bt/min	?
Ralph	140 bt/min	?

12. A male subject performed a submaximal cycle test. Use the single HR-$\dot{V}O_2$ equation and the information provided below to estimate $\dot{V}O_2max$. See Example 12E for assistance.

Test information: body wt = 86 kg
final $\dot{V}O_2$ = 38.30 ml O_2/kg/min
age = 25
HRmax = 195 bt/min
final HR = 175 bt/min

13. Use the double HR-$\dot{V}O_2$ equation to estimate $\dot{V}O_2max$ on a submaximal cycle ergometer test.
Mary, age 30, wt 60 kg, performed a submaximal cycle test using the YMCA branching protocol for females (Table 12.3). Mary's HRmax was 190 bt/min. Use Table 12.1 to convert each of the following cycle workloads to ml O_2/kg/min.

Test Results

Stage	HR (bt/min)	Workload	$\dot{V}O_2$ from Table 12.1 (ml O_2/kg/min)
1	104	150 kgm/min	?
2	120	300 kgm/min	?
3	150	600 kgm/min	?

Double HR-$\dot{V}O_2$ Equation

$$\dot{V}O_2max = (\text{2nd } \dot{V}O_2) + \left[\left(\frac{\text{2nd } \dot{V}O_2 - \text{1st } \dot{V}O_2}{\text{2nd HR} - \text{1st HR}}\right) \times (\text{HRmax} - \text{2nd HR})\right]$$

14. The following subjects performed submaximal exercise tests on a TM. Use the information provided and the double HR-$\dot{V}O_2$ equation to calculate each subject's estimated $\dot{V}O_2max$ in the units ml O_2/kg/min. Do not round off your numbers until the final answer.

	(ml O_2/kg/min)			(bt/min)	
Name	2nd $\dot{V}O_2$	1st $\dot{V}O_2$	2nd HR	1st HR	HRmax
Peter	22	17	130	116	190
Paul	26	23	142	124	182
Mary	25	20	150	128	174

15. Use the information provided for each subject to estimate $\dot{V}O_2max$ using the THR-$\dot{V}O_2$ equation. All subjects achieved their 220 − age × .85% THR (Karvonen method).

    Use Table 12.1 to convert kp workloads to ml O_2/kg/min, relative.

Name	wt (kg)	Final workload	Final $\dot{V}O_2$
George	70	3 kp	?
Alice	80	4 kp	?
Paul	86	3.5 kp	?

THR-$\dot{V}O_2$ Equation

$$\text{Estimated } \dot{V}O_2max = \text{final } \dot{V}O_2 \times 1.174$$

16. The following subjects completed a submaximal exercise test on a treadmill. All achieved their 220 − age × .85% THR (Karvonen method). Calculate each subject's estimated $\dot{V}O_2max$.

Name	Final $\dot{V}O_2$ (ml O_2/kg/min)
Tom	30
Richard	26
Jane	23

17. Kathy is performing a submaximal cycle test using the YMCA branching protocol for females from Table 12.3. Use the following heart rates to determine the correct series of workloads. Try first before looking at the answer.

	HR at end of workload	kgm/min
1st workload □	106	150 (.5 kp)
2nd workload □	120 →	?
3rd workload □	not needed →	?

18. Listed are male subjects who are performing submaximal cycle tests using the YMCA protocol for males, Table 12.2. Determine the next workload for each subject based upon heart rate at the end of each workload stage.

Name	1st workload/HR	2nd workload/HR	3rd workload
Mike	1 kp/94 bt/min	?/140 bt/min	?
Jay	1 kp/110 bt/min	?/146 bt/min	?
Sam	1 kp/88 bt/min	?/118 bt/min	?

Chapter 12 Answers to Practice Problems

1. Completed table:

kp	kgm/min	wt (kg)	ml O_2/min	ml O_2/kg/min	METs
1	300	60	810	13.5	3.8
2	600	80	1,480	18.5	5.3
3.5	1,050	86	2,401	28.0	8.0

2. Jeff's estimated $\dot{V}O_2max$ = 44 ml O_2/kg/min, 12.6 METs.

3. Susan's $\dot{V}O_2max = \frac{900\ \cancel{kgm}}{min} \times \frac{2\ ml\ O_2}{\cancel{kgm}} + 64\ \cancel{kg} \times \frac{3.5\ ml\ O_2}{\cancel{kg}/min}$

$$\dot{V}O_2max = \frac{1{,}800\ ml\ O_2}{min} + \frac{224\ ml\ O_2}{min}$$

$$\dot{V}O_2max = \frac{2{,}024\ ml\ O_2}{min}\ \text{(absolute } \dot{V}O_2\text{)}$$

$$\dot{V}O_2max = 31.63\ ml\ O_2/kg/min\ \text{(relative } \dot{V}O_2\text{)}$$

Note: To determine Susan's estimated $\dot{V}O_2$ we used 2 ml O_2/kgm in the cycle equation. As you can see in Table 12.1, the 2 ml O_2/kgm becomes slightly larger starting at 1,200 kgm/min, which is 2.09 ml O_2/kgm.

4. YMCA cycle test with Alexis

   (a) 450 kgm/min and 1.5 kp

   (b) Correct pedaling rate, 50 rev/min

   (c) 220 − 32 = 188 bt/min = age-predicted HRmax

5. David's predicted maximal workload = 3.5 kp (220 − age 40 = 180 bt/min).

   $\dot{V}O_2max$ = 2.4 L O_2/min
   = 2,401 ml O_2/min
   = 28.0 ml O_2/kg/min (8 METs), rounded off to the nearest whole number

6. $\dot{V}O_2$ from percent grade and speed

Treadmill setting	$\dot{V}O_2$ (ml O_2/kg/min)
2% and 3 mph	14.43
4% and 3.4 mph	19.19
0% (flat) and 187.60 m/min	41.02

7. Lisa's results:

Stage	$\dot{V}O_2$ (ml O_2/kg/min)
1	16.30
2	24.67
3	35.57

   Lisa's predicted $\dot{V}O_2max$ = about 46 to 48 ml O_2/kg/min

8. Mr. Martens' stepping results:

Stage	$\dot{V}O_2$ (ml O_2/kg/min)
1	17.12
2	27.82
3	38.52

Mr. Martens' predicted $\dot{V}O_2max$ = about 50 ml O_2/kg/min (14.3 METs)

9. Determine THR:

Name	THR
John	173
Karen	157
Cliff	153

10. Holly's 3-min step test $\dot{V}O_2max$ values

Test	1-min HR (bt/min)	Est. $\dot{V}O_2max$ (ml O_2/kg/min)
#1	176	33.30
#2	160	36.23

11. Tom and Ralph's $\dot{V}O_2max$ from their step tests

Name	VO_2 (ml O_2/kg/min)
Tom	46.65
Ralph	52.53

12. Single HR-$\dot{V}O_2$ equation, male, estimated $\dot{V}O_2max$

$\dot{V}O_2max$ = 38.30 ml O_2/kg/min $\times$ 1.1754385

$\dot{V}O_2max$ = 45.02 ml O_2/kg/min

13. Mary's cycle test. Double HR-$\dot{V}O_2$ equation

{Stage 2 is the 1st $\dot{V}O_2$ = 13.5 ml O_2/kg/min.
Stage 2 is also the 1st HR = 120 bt/min.

{Stage 3 is the 2nd $\dot{V}O_2$ = 23.5 ml O_2/kg/min.
Stage 3 is the 2nd HR = 150 bt/min.

Remember, you must use HRs that are at or between 115 bt/min and 150 bt/min.

Est. $\dot{V}O_2max$ = 23.5 + (.333333 $\times$ 40)
Est. $\dot{V}O_2max$ = 36.83 ml O_2/kg/min

14. Double HR-$\dot{V}O_2$ equation

Name	Est. $\dot{V}O_2max$
Peter	43.42 ml O_2/kg/min
Paul	32.67 ml O_2/kg/min
Mary	30.45 ml O_2/kg/min

15. Cycle test. THR-$\dot{V}O_2$ equation

Name	ml O_2/kg/min		Constant		ml O_2/kg/min
George	29.2	×	1.174	=	$\dot{V}O_2$max of 34.28
Alice	34.9	×	1.174	=	$\dot{V}O_2$max of 40.97
Paul	28.0	×	1.174	=	$\dot{V}O_2$max of 32.87

16. THR-$\dot{V}O_2$ equation

Name	$\dot{V}O_2$max (ml O_2/kg/min)
Tom	35.22
Richard	30.52
Jane	27.00

17. Kathy's test

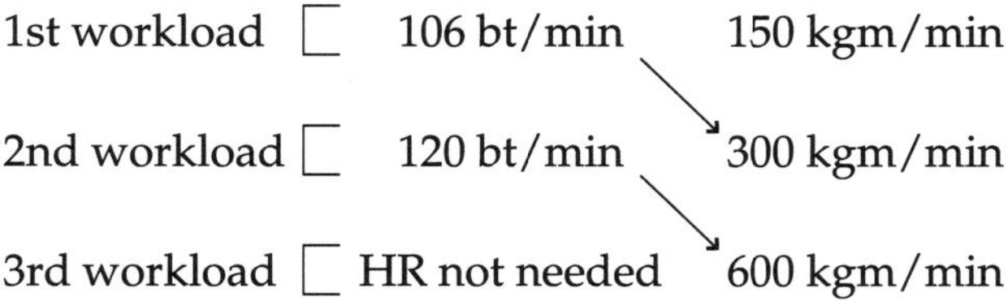

18. YMCA male cycle protocol

Name	1st workload/HR	2nd workload/HR	3rd workload
Mike	1 kp/94	2.5 kp/140	3.0 kp
Jay	1 kp/110	2.0 kp/146	2.5 kp
Sam	1 kp/88	3.0 kp/118	4.5 kp

13 Nutrition Math

Major Concepts

The kilocalorie

Calculations with the three energy nutrients

Calculating ideal body weight

Protein requirements

Calculating total $\dot{V}O_2$, kgm/min, Watts, and METs from kcal/min

Respiratory quotient (RQ) and respiratory gas exchange ratio (R)

Probably you already realize how important nutrition and nutrition-related calculations are in the weight control and disease prevention activities that take place in health and fitness centers.

Of the six nutrients, carbohydrates, fats, and protein are considered the energy nutrients. Each releases measured amounts of energy when digested and metabolized; *Calorie* (kcal) is the term used for this energy. This chapter shows you how to calculate the energy content of food.

One kilocalorie (kcal) or *Calorie* (with a capital C) is equal to 1,000 *calories* (with a small *c*). Food energy is measured in *kcal,* sometimes pronounced *KAY-calories.* Most people, even nutritionists, speak of these units as calories, but on paper and in the scientific community *kcal* is the accepted terminology. To be precise, a kcal, or Calorie, is the amount of heat energy required to raise 1 kilogram of water 1 °C. A calorie, then, is the amount of heat energy required to raise 1 gram of water 1 °C.

The Energy Nutrients

Each energy nutrient (and alcohol) releases the following amount of energy per gram of food weight:

- Carbohydrate = 4 kcal/g
- Protein = 4 kcal/g
- Fats = 9 kcal/g
- Alcohol = 7 kcal/g

(Memorize that list; you will be glad you did.)

Fats, at 9 kcal per gram, contain more than twice the amount of energy found in carbohydrates and proteins, while alcohol, at 7 kcal per gram, contains almost twice the amount. It is easy to see that by simply reducing the intake of fats, a person can significantly reduce the intake of total kcals.

Although alcohol is not considered a nutrient, we cannot forget about its kcal content. Alcohol is metabolized, as are the three energy nutrients, to yield energy. When kcals are consumed in excess of daily energy expenditure, the energy is converted into triglycerides, which are stored as adipose (body fat) tissue.

The following section contains a series of nutrition-related math examples; the calculations are of the type that you might find on exercise physiology exams or use at work.

Determining the Energy Content of Food

Food sources contain vitamins, minerals, water, and the three energy nutrients carbohydrates, fat, and protein. Using the constants for kcal/g of nutrients, you can determine the calorie content of food given its nutrient composition.

Example 13A

Determine the kcal content per gram of weight of one potato. An average potato has 3 g of protein, 21 g of carbohydrates, and a trace of fat (can be ignored). What is the kcal content?

Step 1: Determine kcals from protein.

$$\text{kcal from protein} = 3\ \text{g}\ \cancel{\text{protein}} \times \frac{4\ \text{kcal}}{1\ \text{g}\ \cancel{\text{protein}}} = 12\ \text{kcal}$$

Step 2: Determine kcals from carbohydrates.

$$\text{kcal from carb} = 21\ \cancel{\text{g carb}} \times \frac{4\ \text{kcal}}{\cancel{\text{g carb}}} = 84\ \text{kcal}$$

Step 3: Add kcals.

$$12 + 84 = 96\ \text{kcal in the potato}$$

The number of kcal per gram of potato can be calculated if you know the potato's weight. If the average potato weighs 3.5 oz and contains 96 kcal, then the kcal/g would be:

$$3.5\ \cancel{\text{oz}}\ \text{potato} \times \frac{28\ \text{g}}{1\ \cancel{\text{oz}}} = 98\ \text{g potato}$$

$$\frac{96\ \text{kcal}}{98\ \text{g potato}} = .98\ \text{kcal/g of potato (or approximately 1 kcal/1 g potato)}$$

A similar approach can be used to estimate the number of kcal in a food item based on the nutrient content listed on the food label.

Example 13B

Calculate the kcal/g value of one bagel. A 2-oz bagel contains 6 g protein, 2 g fat, and 28 g carbohydrate. How many total kcal are in the bagel? How many kcal/g?

Step 1: Find kcal from protein.

$$\text{kcal protein} = 6\ \cancel{\text{g}}\ \text{protein} \times \frac{4\ \text{kcal}}{\cancel{\text{g}}} = 24\ \text{kcal protein}$$

Step 2: Find kcal from fat.

$$\text{kcal fat} = 2\ \cancel{\text{g}}\ \text{fat} \times \frac{9\ \text{kcal}}{\cancel{\text{g}}} = 18\ \text{kcal fat}$$

Step 3: Find kcal from carbohydrates.

$$\text{kcal carb} = 28\ \cancel{\text{g}}\ \text{carb} \times \frac{4\ \text{kcal}}{\cancel{\text{g}}} = 112\ \text{kcal carb}$$

Step 4: Combine kcals.

$$24\ \text{kcal} + 18\ \text{kcal} + 112\ \text{kcal} = 154\ \text{kcal in a 2-oz bagel}$$

Step 5: Convert weight in 2 oz to g and divide to find kcal/g.

$$2\ \cancel{\text{oz}}\ \text{bagel} \times \frac{28\ \text{g}}{1\ \cancel{\text{oz}}} = 56\ \text{g bagel}$$

$$\frac{154\ \text{kcal}}{56\ \text{g bagel}} = 2.75\ \text{kcal/g of bagel}$$

Calculating Percent Fat in Food

Low-fat foods are considered more heart healthy than high-fat foods. It is often necessary to calculate the percent of fat in foods.

Example 13C

Determine percentage of fat in a 2-oz bagel. What percentage of the total kcal in the bagel (see Example 13B) is from fat?

The bagel has 18 kcal from fat out of 154 total kcal. Therefore,

$$\frac{18\ \text{kcal fat}}{154\ \text{kcal total}} = 11.69\%$$

or approximately 12% of the kcal in the bagel are from fat.

Calculating Percentage of Daily Food Intake From Fats, Proteins, and Carbohydrates

The American Heart Association (1982, 1988) suggests that of the total daily caloric intake no more than 30% of kcal should come from fats, about 15% of kcal should come from protein, and 55 to 60% should come from carbohydrates. It is often necessary to evaluate an individual's diet to determine either the number of kcal from various sources or the percentages of nutrients within the diet, as in the following examples.

Example 13D

Determine kcal content from each energy nutrient when given the total kcal intake. Frank consumes 3,000 kcal/day. Frank follows the AHA recommendations. How many kcal from each food source is he consuming per day?

Step 1: Multiply kcal from each nutrient by AHA recommended percentages.

3,000 kcal × .30 fat = 900 kcal from fat
3,000 kcal × .15 protein = 450 kcal from protein
3,000 kcal × .55 carb = 1,650 kcal from carb

The total should be 3,000 (because fat, protein, and carbohydrate make up 100% of intake)—if it is not, a math error was made.

It is sometimes useful to ascertain the percentage of the diet that comes from each of the three nutrients when the total caloric intake and the amounts of the nutrients are known.

Example 13E

Determine the percentage of kcal in a subject's daily kcal intake. Roger consumes 3,000 kcal of food per day: 70 g of fat, 450 g of carbohydrate, and 142.5 g of protein.

Step 1: Determine kcal from each food.

70 g fat × 9 kcal = 630 kcal fat
450 g carb × 4 kcal = 1,800 kcal carb
142.5 g pro × 4 kcal = 570 kcal protein

Step 2: Determine the percent from each food.

$$\frac{630 \text{ ~~kcal~~ fat}}{3{,}000 \text{ ~~kcal total~~}} = 21\% \text{ dietary fat}$$

$$\frac{1{,}800 \text{ ~~kcal~~ carb}}{3{,}000 \text{ ~~kcal total~~}} = 60\% \text{ dietary carb}$$

$$\frac{570 \text{ ~~kcal~~ pro}}{3{,}000 \text{ ~~kcal total~~}} = 19\% \text{ dietary protein}$$

100%

Again, if the percentages don't add up to 100%, a math error was made.

Protein Requirements

Protein requirements vary slightly per individual, but there is an RDA (recommended dietary allowance) for the amount of protein needed for good health and disease prevention. Recommended dietary allowances (RDAs) are levels of intake of essential nutrients considered adequate to meet the known nutritional needs of the majority of healthy adults, as stated by the Committee on Dietary Allowances of the Food and Nutrition Board in Washington, DC. There is a separate list of RDAs for children based on age. Note: The *D* within RDA means *dietary*, not *daily*. (Whitney & Hamilton, 1977, p. 40; Worthington-Roberts, 1981). There are two methods for determining a subject's protein requirements (Whitney & Hamilton, 1977, p. 97; McArdle et al., 1994, ch. 3). The first is based upon an individual's present weight. The second is based upon an individual's IBW (ideal body weight). The conversion factor for the requirement based on present weight is .8 g protein/1 kg present wt. The conversion factor for the requirement based on IBW is .8 g protein/ 1 kg of IBW.

You may need to determine protein requirements using the .8 g unit based either on a subject's present weight or on IBW. The following discussion and examples will include both methods.

Example 13F

Determine protein requirements considering total body weight and IBW. Janice has a total body weight of 72 kg. Her ideal body weight is 60 kg. Find her daily protein requirements using both methods.

Step 1: Multiply body wt × conversion factor to find g/day of protein required based on present weight.

72 × .8 g protein/day = 57.6 g protein/day

Step 2: Multiply ideal body wt × conversion factor to find g/day of protein required based on IBW.

60 × .8 g protein/day = 48 g protein/day

Calculating IBW (Ideal Body Weight)

Ideal body weight is a concept used in nutritional calculations such as determination of the protein requirement. An individual's IBW can be defined as the body weight at which the percentage of body fat falls into the recommended ranges based upon age and gender (Lohman, 1981, 1984a, 1984b; Pollock et al., 1978). For adult men, 12%–18% body fat is optimal for good health. For adult women, 16%–25% body fat is optimal.

Example 13G illustrates the concept of ideal body weight.

Example 13G

Determine IBW (ACSM, 1988). Neil weighs 225 lb and his body is about 30% fat. His ideal percentage of body fat is 24%. What is his IBW?

Step 1: Determine fat weight in lb.

225 lb × .30 = 68 lb fat

Step 2: Determine lean weight in pounds (total weight − fat weight = lean weight).

225 lb total
− 68 lb fat
157 lb lean

Step 3: Determine percent of lean desired.

$$\begin{array}{r} 100\ \%\ \text{total} \\ -\ \ 24\ \%\ \text{fat desired} \\ \hline 76\ \%\ \text{lean desired} \end{array}$$

Step 4: Determine IBW based upon desired lean weight.

$$\frac{157\ \text{lb lean}}{.76\ \text{desired lean}} = 206.58\ \text{lb or about } 206\ \text{lb}$$

For Neil to achieve 24% body fat he needs to decrease his body fat so that he drops his body weight from 225 lb to about 206.58 lb.

Converting kcal/min to $\dot{V}O_2$, METs, and Cycle or Treadmill Workloads

Converting kcal/min to $\dot{V}O_2$ and METs and to cycle and treadmill workloads is a fundamental calculation in exercise physiology. You will certainly be required to perform these calculations on exams and on the job. It would be useful for you to memorize the information in this section rather than using it as reference material.

As we saw in previous chapters, a total absolute $\dot{V}O_2$ can be converted into kcal/min. Here we will consider the reverse calculation. From a given kcal/min we can determine a subject's total $\dot{V}O_2$ and METs. From the $\dot{V}O_2$ and METs it is possible to calculate the workloads that will be needed to consume the given kcal/min, as illustrated in Example 13H.

Example 13H

Find workload needed to consume a given kcal/min. We would like Roger to consume 15 kcal/min while riding a stationary cycle.

Step 1: Convert kcal/min to ml O_2/min.

$$\text{kcal/min} \times \text{conversion factor} = \text{absolute } \dot{V}O_2$$

$$\frac{15\ \cancel{\text{kcal}}}{\text{min}} \times \frac{1\ \text{ml}\ O_2}{.005\ \cancel{\text{kcal}}} = \frac{3{,}000\ \text{ml}\ O_2}{\text{min}}$$

Step 2: Roger's weight is 72 kg. Convert the absolute $\dot{V}O_2$ of 3,000 ml O_2/min to a relative $\dot{V}O_2$ and divide the absolute $\dot{V}O_2$ by Roger's weight.

$$\frac{3{,}000\ \text{ml}\ O_2/\text{min}}{72\ \text{kg}} = 41.67\ \text{ml}\ O_2/\text{kg/min}$$

Step 3: Convert ml O_2/kg/min to METs.

$$\frac{41.67\ \cancel{\text{ml}\ O_2/\text{kg/min}}}{1} \times \frac{1\ \text{MET}}{3.5\ \cancel{\text{ml}\ O_2/\text{kg/min}}} = 11.9\ \text{METs}$$

Step 4: Refer back to table 10.2 in Chapter 10 to convert the 41.67 ml O_2/kg/min (11.9 METs) to a cycle workload of kgm/min or Watts. Then use Appendix D to convert the $\dot{V}O_2$ to walking or running speed.

Roger would have to pedal a stationary cycle at a workload of about 1,275 kgm/min or about 212 Watts to consume 15 kcal/min. He'd have to run at just over 7 mph on a level treadmill to consume the same amount of kcal/min.

Respiratory Quotient and Respiratory Gas Exchange Ratio

This section presents the basic mathematical concepts concerning respiratory quotient (RQ) and respiratory gas exchange ratio (R). The information is intended to help you remember and conceptualize the RQ and R equation and the related number values. You will notice that the respiratory gas exchange ratio is abbreviated as RER in some other texts or journal articles. Either abbreviation, R or RER, is acceptable. In this book we use R.

Respiratory quotient is a reflection of the amount of CO_2 produced compared to the amount of O_2 consumed at the tissue level; it represents fuel (substrate) metabolism. RQ is mathematically derived from this equation:

$$RQ = \frac{VCO_2}{VO_2}$$

You'll notice that the *V*s in this equation do not have dots over them. The dot over the *V* indicates *per minute.* In most cases when steady-state CO_2 and O_2 are recorded for RQ, the gases are collected over several minutes.

Each of the energy nutrients—fat, protein, and carbohydrate—requires a different amount of oxygen for metabolism and each produces a different amount of carbon dioxide when metabolized. By analysis of the ratio of the volume of CO_2 produced to the volume of O_2 consumed, the major fuel source that an individual is using for energy can be identified (McArdle et al., 1994). Table 13.1 shows the values representing the metabolic fuel source of each of the energy nutrients.

You can see that the RQ value of .80 represents the metabolism of just protein. The RQ value of .82 to .84 represents a mixture of 40% fuel from fat and 60% from carbohydrate. Protein is usually not considered within the RQ at this point because protein plays such a small part in energy production at rest or during submaximal steady-state workloads.

The RQ values measured during rest and steady-state submaximal exercise most often do not reflect metabolism of a pure food source, but rather a mixture of fat and carbohydrate, with an RQ range between .70 and 1.0. An RQ value nearing 1.00 indicates a fuel source mixture of mostly carbohydrate. An RQ nearing .70 is an indicator that fats are being metabolized as the predominant fuel source.

Table 13.1 RQ Values Representing Metabolic Fuel Source

Food source	**RQ = VCO_2/VO_2**
Pure carbohydrates	1.00
Pure protein	.80
Pure fat	.70
Mixed diet	.82–.84

Respiratory gas exchange ratio is calculated in exactly the same way that RQ is. R, however, is measured at the lung level, not the tissue level, and this term is used when exercise intensity is increasing rapidly up to the point of $\dot{V}O_2max$. R is measured during non-steady-state exercise during intense effort. Values of 1.00 to 1.20 are seen during maximal effort graded exercise testing when subjects reach their true $\dot{V}O_2max$ while being tested on a treadmill.

As an individual approaches $\dot{V}O_2max$ during a graded exercise test, O_2 consumption begins to level off in the presence of increasing workloads. CO_2 production continues to increase. The increasing CO_2 production during intensive exercise, a response to lactate buffering, can no longer be attributed to cellular-level substrate metabolism. At this point R often becomes 1.00 or greater. An R of 1.00, often referred to as "unity" in exercise physiology literature, means that O_2 uptake is equal to CO_2 production. An R of 1.00 or greater, and the leveling off of O_2 consumption, are both helpful pieces of additional information to support the attainment of $\dot{V}O_2max$.

Example 131

Determine RQ and fuel source. A sedentary subject is resting quietly. Open-circuit spirometry shows that he produced 2,000 ml CO_2 and that he consumed 2,800 ml of O_2. Determine RQ and the major fuel source.

Remember, the O_2 goes on the bottom of the equation!

Step 1: Fill in the equation and divide.

$$RQ = \frac{VCO_2}{VO_2} = \frac{2{,}000 \cancel{\text{ml } CO_2}}{2{,}800 \cancel{\text{ml } O_2}} = .71$$

Step 2: Check Table 13.1 for fuel source. With an RQ of .71, fat is the major fuel source.

The practice problems will give you more exposure to RQ and R calculations.

Summary

When metabolized, each of the energy nutrients releases a specific amount of energy in the form of kcal. Using the math provided within this chapter you can determine the percentage of each of the energy nutrients contained within a diet, meal, or single food item along with the number of kcals provided by carbohydrates, fats, or proteins. Protein requirements can also be determined for an individual on the basis of total body weight or ideal body weight. The desired kcal/min to be consumed during exercise can be converted into the correct $\dot{V}O_2$ or workloads for a specific ergometer.

RQ (respiratory quotient) and R (respiratory gas exchange ratio) were also discussed in this chapter. RQ represents CO_2/O_2 values at the cellular level during rest or steady-state submaximal exercise, and R represents CO_2/O_2 values at the lung level.

Chapter 13 Practice Problems

If you experience difficulty arriving at a reasonable answer to any of the following problems, try not to go immediately to the answer page. Instead, work the problem again, trying different math combinations.

Conversion factor for converting oz to g or vice versa:

$$\frac{1\text{ oz}}{28\text{ g}} \text{ or } \frac{28\text{ g}}{1\text{ oz}}$$

1. Convert the following list of oz to g.

   (a) 32 oz of carrots

   (b) 10 oz of roasted peanuts

2. Convert the following to oz.

   (a) 85 g of hamburger (one patty)

   (b) 56 g hot dog (one baseball park, regulation, 5-in hot dog)

3. Determine the kcal content of the following.

   (a) 150 g of carb

   (b) 75 g of protein

4. Analyze the kcal content in one loaf of wheat bread. One loaf contains 40 g of protein, 10 g of fat, and 236 g of carb.

   (a) Determine total kcal content

   (b) This loaf contain 20 slices. How many kcals are in each slice?

5. A noon meal for Julie includes a variety of food items containing the following proportions of protein, fat, and carb: 50 g of protein, 35 g of fat, and 255 g of carb.

   (a) Determine the total kcal content of Julie's noon meal.

   (b) Determine the percentage of total kcal that comes from fat.

6. John consumes the following in one day: 102 g of protein, 70 g of fat, and 510 g of carb.

   (a) Determine John's total kcal consumption in one day.

   (b) Determine the percentage of kcal that comes from protein, fat, and carb.

   (c) Add together the percentages. Do they add up to 100%?

7. Tom consumes about 3,200 kcal each day during his training season. His dietary selection is 30% from fats, 15% from protein sources, and 55% from carbohydrate sources. Find the kcal intake from each of these food sources.

8. What is the daily protein requirement of a man who is at his IBW of 160 lb? First, convert lb to kg.

9. Determine Joe's IBW. He is 28 and weighs 235 lb. His present body composition is 25% fat, and his desired body composition is 18% fat, ? % lean.

10. Convert the following to kcal/min. Subject's weight = 72 kg.

    (a) $\frac{2{,}400\text{ ml }O_2}{\text{min}}$

    (b) 3,800 ml O_2/min

(c) $\frac{61.12 \text{ ml } O_2}{\text{kg/min}}$

(d) 50 ml O2/kg/min

11. Convert the following kcal/min to absolute $\dot{V}O_2$ values.

(a) $\frac{8 \text{ kcal}}{\text{min}}$

(b) 24 kcal/min

12. Kenneth weighs 68 kg. Find his absolute $\dot{V}O_2$, relative $\dot{V}O_2$, and MET level, given 14 kcal/min = energy expenditure.

13. You would like to expend 13.5 kcal/min while riding a cycle ergometer. Your weight is 82 kg. Determine the desired cycle workload in kgm/min and Watts for the cycle ergometer. Hint: Review the cycle equation in chapter 10. You may want to use Tables 10.1 and 10.2.

14. Find jogging speed in the units m/min and mph for the treadmill to satisfy the energy expenditure of 13 kcal/min. Subject's weight = 82 kg.

Hint: Use the horizontal $\dot{V}O_2$ component for running (level) in chapter 9.

15. Determine RQ and the fuel source from the following values that were obtained (collected) during steady-state submaximal cycling.

VO_2 = 2,125 ml O_2
VCO_2 = 1,785 ml CO_2

16. Determine respiratory quotient (RQ) and the fuel source. Subject is resting; VCO_2 = 4 L CO_2 produced and VO_2 = 4 L O_2 consumed.

Chapter 13 Answers to Practice Problems

1. (a) $32 \not{oz} \times \frac{28 \text{ g}}{1 \not{oz}}$ = 896 g of carrots, about 8 cups grated carrots

(b) 280 g of roasted peanuts (about 2 cups)

2. (a) 3.04 oz hamburger patty

(b) 2 oz = one hot dog

3. $150 \text{ g carb} \times \frac{4 \text{ kcal}}{1 \text{ g carb}} = 600 \text{ kcal}$

(b) $75 \text{ g protein} \times \frac{4 \text{ kcal}}{1 \text{ g protein}} = 300 \text{ kcal}$

4. (a)

160 kcal protein
90 kcal fat
\+ 944 kcal carb

1,194 total kcal per loaf of wheat bread

(b) $\frac{1{,}194 \text{ kcal}}{\cancel{\text{one loaf}}} \times \frac{\cancel{\text{one loaf}}}{20 \text{ slices}} = \frac{59.7 \text{ kcal}}{\text{slice}}$

The units kcal and slice remain uncanceled, leaving kcal/slice as the answer.

5. 1,535 total kcal, $\frac{315 \cancel{\text{kcal}}}{1{,}535 \cancel{\text{kcal}}}$ = approx. 20% of the total kcal from fat

6. 3,078 total kcal

$$\frac{408 \cancel{\text{kcal}}}{3{,}078 \cancel{\text{kcal}}} = 13.26\% \text{ from protein}$$

$$\frac{630 \cancel{\text{kcal}}}{3{,}078 \cancel{\text{kcal}}} = 20.47\% \text{ from fat}$$

$$\frac{2{,}040 \cancel{\text{kcal}}}{3{,}078 \cancel{\text{kcal}}} = 66.28\% \text{ from carbs}$$

7.

$$\frac{3{,}200 \text{ kcal}}{\text{day}} \times .30 \text{ fat} = \frac{960 \text{ kcal fat}}{\text{day}}$$

$$\frac{3{,}200 \text{ kcal}}{\text{day}} \times .15 \text{ protein} = \frac{480 \text{ kcal protein}}{\text{day}}$$

$$\frac{3{,}200 \text{ kcal}}{\text{day}} \times .55 \text{ carb} = \frac{1{,}760 \text{ kcal carb}}{\text{day}}$$

3,200 kcal total

8. Man with weight of 160 lb

$$160 \cancel{\text{lb}} \times \frac{1 \text{ kg}}{2.2 \cancel{\text{lb}}} = 73 \text{ kg}$$

$$73 \cancel{\text{kg}} \times \frac{.8 \text{ g protein}}{1 \cancel{\text{kg}}} = 58.4 \text{ g protein required per day}$$

9. Joe, age 28

Step 1: 235 lb × .25 fat = 58.75 lb fat   18% fat desired
82% lean desired

Step 2: 235.00 lb total
− 58.75 lb fat
176.25 lb lean

Step 3: $\frac{176.25 \text{ lb lean}}{.82 \text{ lean desired}} = \frac{214.93 \text{ lb}}{\text{desired}}$ = IBW = 215 lb

10. Subject, weight of 72 kg

(a) $\frac{2{,}400 \cancel{\text{ml } O_2}}{\text{min}} \times \frac{.005 \text{ kcal}}{1 \cancel{\text{ml } O_2}} = \frac{12 \text{ kcal}}{\text{min}}$

(b) 19 kcal/min

(c) $\frac{61.12 \text{ ml } O_2}{\cancel{\text{kg}}/\text{min}} \times \frac{72 \cancel{\text{kg}}}{1} = \frac{4{,}400 \text{ ml } O_2}{\text{min}}$

$\frac{4{,}400 \cancel{\text{ml } O_2}}{\text{min}} \times \frac{.005 \text{ kcal}}{1 \cancel{\text{ml } O_2}} = \frac{22 \text{ kcal}}{\text{min}}$

(d) 18 kcal/min

11. Converting kcal/min to absolute $\dot{V}O_2$

(a) $\frac{8\ \text{kcal}}{\text{min}} \times \frac{1\ \text{ml}\ O_2}{.005\ \text{kcal}} = \frac{1{,}600\ \text{ml}\ O_2}{\text{min}}$

(b) $\frac{4{,}800\ \text{ml}\ O_2}{\text{min}} = \frac{4.8\ \text{L}\ O_2}{\text{min}}$

12. Absolute $\dot{V}O_2 = \frac{2{,}800\ \text{ml}\ O_2}{\text{min}}$

Relative $\dot{V}O_2$ = 41.176 ml O_2/kg/min

METs = 11.76 METs

13. Review the cycle equation in chapter 10.

Step 1: Convert kcal to ml O_2.

$$13.5\ \text{kcal} \times \frac{\text{ml}\ O_2}{.005\ \text{kcal}} = 2{,}700\ \text{ml}\ O_2\ (\text{total}\ \dot{V}O_2)$$

Step 2: Determine resting $\dot{V}O_2$ component of cycle equation using the subject's body weight.

$$\frac{3.5\ \text{ml}\ O_2}{\text{kg/min}} \times \frac{82\ \text{kg}}{1} = 287\ \text{ml}\ O_2/\text{min}$$

Step 3: We are now working the cycle equation in reverse. Subtract the resting component for the total $\dot{V}O_2$, leaving the resistive $\dot{V}O_2$ component.

$$\text{Total absolute}\ \dot{V}O_2 = \frac{2{,}700\ \text{ml}\ O_2}{\text{min}} - \frac{287\ \text{ml}\ O_2}{\text{min}} = \frac{2{,}413\ \text{ml}\ O_2}{\text{min}}$$

Step 4: Divide the resistive $\dot{V}O_2$ component by 2 ml O_2 to arrive at cycle resistance.

$$\text{Workload for cycle} = \frac{2{,}413\ \text{ml}\ O_2}{\text{min}} \times \frac{\text{kgm}}{2\ \text{ml}\ O_2} = \frac{1{,}206.5\ \text{kgm}}{\text{min}}$$

Step 5: Convert to Watts by dividing by 6.

$\frac{1\ \text{Watt}}{6\ \text{kgm/min}}$ is the conversion factor.

$$1{,}206.5\ \text{kgm/min} \times \frac{1\ \text{Watt}}{6\ \text{kgm/min}} = 201.08\ \text{Watts}$$

For setting the resistance on the cycle, these answers can be rounded off to 1,200 kgm/min and 200 Watts. Now, refer to table 10.1 (chapter 10). The value of 200 Watts on the cycle can be 2 kp at 100 rev/min or 4 kp at 50 rev/min to expend 13.5 kcal/min.

Extra information: At the above cycle workload it would take you 4.42 min to expend the kcal energy in one slice of wheat bread, i.e., from problem 4,

$$\frac{59.7\ \text{kcal}}{\text{slice}} \times \frac{\text{min}}{13.5\ \text{kcal}} = \frac{4.42\ \text{min}}{\text{slice}}.$$

14. Total absolute $\dot{V}O_2$ = 2,600 ml O_2/min

Total relative $\dot{V}O_2$ = 31.7 ml O_2/kg/min

(Total Relative $\dot{V}O_2$) − (Rest $\dot{V}O_2$) = (Horiz $\dot{V}O_2$)

31.7 ml O_2/kg/min − 3.5 ml O_2/kg/min = 28.2 ml O_2/kg/min

Jogging speed:

$$28.2\ \cancel{\text{ml } O_2/\text{kg}/\text{min}} \times \frac{\text{m/min}}{0.2\ \cancel{\text{ml } O_2/\text{kg}/\text{min}}} = 141.0\ \text{m/min}$$

$$141.0\ \cancel{\text{m/min}} \times \frac{1\ \text{mph}}{26.8\ \cancel{\text{m/min}}} = 5.26\ \text{mph}$$

15. $$\text{RQ} = \frac{VCO_2}{VO_2} = \frac{1{,}785\ \cancel{\text{ml } CO_2}}{2{,}125\ \cancel{\text{ml } O_2}} = .84 = \text{mixed diet}$$

16. $$\frac{4\ \cancel{\text{L } CO_2}}{4\ \cancel{\text{L } O_2}} = 1.00 = \text{''unity,'' an all-carb diet}$$

A Abbreviations

Units of Measure

g—gram
J—joule
kcal—kilocalorie
kgm—kilogram-meter
km—kilometer
kpm—kilopond-meter
m—meter
MET—metabolic equivalent
N—newton
rev/min—revolutions per minute
sec—second
W—Watts

Terminology

a-$\bar{v}$ O_2 diff—arterial-mixed venous oxygen difference
BMR—basal metabolic rate
BP—blood pressure
DBP—diastolic blood pressure
DS—dead space
ECG—electrocardiography (also written as EKG)
EF—ejection fraction
EDV—end diastolic volume
ESV—end systolic volume
FEO_2—fractional (percentage) of oxygen expired
FIO_2—fractional (percentage) of oxygen inhaled
$FECO_2$—fractional (percentage) of carbon dioxide expired
$FICO_2$—fractional (percentage) of carbon dioxide inhaled
FIN_2—fraction of nitrogen in inhaled air

FEN_2—fraction of nitrogen in exhaled air
F—fractional
f—frequency; most often associated with rate or frequency of breathing
GXT—graded exercise test
HR—heart rate
HRR—heart rate reserve
LVD—left ventricular dysfunction
MAP—mean arterial pressure
mmHg—millimeters of mercury
$\dot{Q}$—cardiac output
REE—resting energy expenditure
RPE—rated perceived exertion
RQ—respiratory quotient
R—RER; respiratory gas exchange ratio
SBP—systolic blood pressure
SV—stroke volume
THR—target heart rate or training heart rate
TM—treadmill
TV—tidal volume
V—total volume of gas or air
$\dot{V}$—volume of gas or air per minute, pronounced "v-dot"
$\dot{V}A$—alveolar ventilation per minute
$\dot{V}E$—minute ventilation per minute
$\dot{V}O_2$—volume of oxygen consumed per minute, pronounced "v-dot O_2"
$\dot{V}CO_2$—volume of carbon dioxide exhaled per minute, pronounced "v-dot CO_2"
$\dot{V}O_2max$—maximal volume of oxygen uptake per minute
VC—vital capacity

B Conversion Factors

Distances

1 ft = 12 in
1 yd = 3 ft
1 mile = 5,280 ft
1 mile = 1,760 yd
1 m = 100 cm
1 km = 1,000 m
1 in = 2.54 cm
1 yd = .9144 m
1 mile = 1.62 km
1 m = 39.37 in
1 m = 3.28 ft
1 km = 1,093.6 yd
1 km = .62 miles

Speeds

1 mph = 1.47 ft/sec
1 mph = 88 ft/min
60 mph = 88 ft/sec
1 km/hr = .28 m/sec
1 km/hr = 16.7 m/min
1 mph = .45 m/sec
1 mph = 26.8 m/min
1 mph = 1.62 km/hr
1 km/hr = .62 mph
1 km/hr = .91 ft/sec

Weights

1 oz = 28 g
1 lb = 454 g
1 g = 1,000 mg
1 kg = 1,000 g
1 kg = 1 kp
1 kg = 2.2 lb
1 kg = 9.8 N

Volumes (O_2, CO_2, N_2, or Blood)

1 oz = 29.57 ml
1 quart = 1.11 L
1 dl = 100 ml
1 L = 1,000 ml

Work Units

1 kcal = 426.8 kgm
.005 kcal = 1 ml O_2
5 kcal = 1 L O_2
1 kgm = 1.8 ml O_2
1 kcal/kg/hr = 1 MET
1.8 ml O_2/kg/in = 1 kgm/min (for leg ergometer only)
1 kg body wt/m/min = 1.8 ml O_2 (for leg ergometer only)

Workload Units

1 Watt = 6.0 kgm/min
1 MET = 3.5 ml O_2/kg/min
1 kgm/min = .1635 Watts
1.8 ml O_2/kg/min = 1 m/min
1 HP = 746 Watts
1 L O_2/min = 5 kcal/min
2 ml O_2 = 1 kgm (for leg ergometers)
3 ml O_2 = 1 kgm (for arm ergometers)
0.35 ml O_2/kg/min = 1 step/min (for bench stepping)
0.1 ml O_2/kg/min = 1 m/min (for walking)
0.2 ml O_2/kg/min = 1 m/min (for running)

Nutrition Units

4 kcal = 1 g protein
9 kcal = 1 g fat
4 kcal = 1 g carb
7 kcal = 1 g alcohol
28 g = 1 oz
.005 kcal = 1 ml O_2

C Table of Approximate Metabolic Values

Term	Unit	Average adult: Pre-training	Average adult: Post-training	Endurance athlete
Heart rate (rest)*	bt/min	74	56	40
Heart rate (max)*	bt/min	185	180	170
Stroke volume (rest)	ml/bt	70	80	125
Stroke volume (max)	ml/bt	120	140	200
$\dot{Q}$ (rest)	L/min	4.6	4.8	4.5
$\dot{Q}$ (max)	L/min	22.2	25.6	34.8
Heart volume (size of heart)	ml	750	820	1200
Blood volume (body)	L	4.7	5.1	6.0
$\dot{V}E$ (rest)	L air/min	7	6	6
$\dot{V}E$ (max)	L air/min	110	135	190
f (rest)	breaths/min	14	12	12
f (max)	breaths/min	40	45	55
TV(rest)	ml air/breath	500	500	500
TV(max)	ml air/breath	2750	3000	3500
a-$\bar{v}$ O_2 diff (rest)	ml O_2/100 ml blood	6	6	6
a-$\bar{v}$ O_2 diff (max)	ml O_2/100 ml blood	14.5	15	16
$\dot{V}O_2$ (rest)	ml O_2/kg/min	3.5	3.7	4.0
$\dot{V}O_2$ (max)	ml O_2/kg/min	40	50	75
Blood lactate (rest)	mg/100 ml blood	10	10	10
Blood lactate (max)	mg/100 ml blood	110	125	185

*rest = at or near 1 MET; max = at or near $\dot{V}O_2$max.

D Table of $\dot{V}O_2$ From Walking and Running Equations

Walking speeds, 1.7 to 4.2 mph

Speed (mph) **% grade**	**1.7** **45.56**	**2.0** **53.60**	**2.5** **67.00**	**3.0** **80.40**	**3.3** **88.44**	**3.4** **91.12**	**3.75** **100.5**	**4.0** **107.5**	**4.2** **112.56**	**mph** **m/min**
0	8.10	8.86	10.20	11.54	12.34	12.61	13.55	14.22	14.76	
2	9.74	10.79	13.08	14.43	15.53	15.89	17.17	18.08	18.81	
2.5	10.15	11.27	13.22	15.16	16.32	16.71	18.07	19.04	19.82	
4	11.38	12.72	15.02	17.33	18.71	19.19	20.79	21.94	22.86	
6	13.02	14.65	17.44	20.22	21.90	22.45	24.40	25.80	26.92	
8	14.66	16.58	19.85	23.12	25.10	25.73	28.02	29.66	30.97	
10	16.30	18.51	22.26	26.01	28.26	29.01	31.64	33.54	35.02	
12	17.94	20.44	24.67	28.91	31.45	32.29	35.26	37.38	39.07	
14	19.58	22.37	27.08	31.80	34.63	35.57	38.88	41.23	43.12	
16	21.22	24.30	29.50	34.70	37.81	38.85	42.50	45.10	47.18	
18	22.86	26.23	31.91	37.59	41.00	42.13	46.11	48.95	51.23	
20	24.50	28.16	34.32	40.48	44.18	45.42	49.73	52.81	55.28	

Running speeds, 5.0 to 12 mph

Speed (mph) **% grade**	**5.0** **134**	**5.5** **147.40**	**6.0** **160.80**	**7.0** **187.60**	**8.0** **214.40**	**9.0** **241.20**	**10** **268.00**	**11** **294.80**	**12** **321.60**	**mph** **m/min**
0	30.30	32.98	35.66	41.02	46.38	51.74	57.10	62.46	67.82	
2	32.71	35.63	38.55	44.40	50.24	56.08	61.92	67.77	73.61	
4	35.12	38.29	41.45	47.77	54.10	60.42	66.75	73.07	79.40	
6	37.54	40.94	44.34	51.22	58.02	64.83	71.64	78.44	85.25	
8	39.95	43.59	47.24	54.53	61.82	69.12	76.40	83.69	90.98	

10	42.36	46.25	50.13	57.90	65.68	73.45	81.22	88.99	96.76
12	44.77	48.90	53.03	61.28	69.52	77.76	86.00	94.25	102.49
14	47.18	51.55	55.92	64.66	73.39	82.13	90.87	99.60	108.34
16	49.60	54.20	58.82	68.03	77.25	86.47	95.69	104.91	114.13
18	52.01	56.86	61.71	71.41	81.11	90.81	100.52	110.22	119.92
20	54.42	59.51	64.60	74.79	84.98	95.16	105.34	115.52	125.71

E Metabolic Equations

Temperature Conversion, Chapter 2

$$F^\circ = (1.8 \times C^\circ) + 32 \qquad C^\circ = \frac{(F^\circ - 32)}{1.8}$$

Cardiovascular Dynamics, Chapter 4

Solving for $\dot{V}O_2$

$$\dot{V}O_2 = \dot{Q} \times a\text{–}\bar{v}\ O_2\ \text{diff}$$

$$\dot{V}O_2 = SV \times HR \times a\text{–}\bar{v}\ O_2\ \text{diff}$$

$$\dot{V}O_2 = EDV \times EF \times HR \times a\text{–}\bar{v}\ O_2\ \text{diff}$$

Fick equation

Solving for SV or EF

$$SV = EDV \times EF \quad \text{or} \quad \frac{SV}{EDV} = EF \quad \text{or} \quad SV = EDV - ESV$$

Solving for a-$\bar{v}$ O2 difference

a-$\bar{v}$ O_2 diff

= ml O_2/100 ml arterial blood minus ml O_2/100 ml mixed venous blood

Solving for Cardiac Output ($\dot{Q}$)

$$\dot{Q} = \frac{\dot{V}O_2}{a\text{-}\bar{v}\ O_2\ \text{diff}} \text{ or } \dot{Q} = SV \times HR$$

O_2 Pulse Equations

$$O_2\ \text{Pulse} = \frac{\dot{V}O_2}{HR}$$

$$O_2\ \text{Pulse} = \frac{\dot{Q} \times a-\bar{v}\ O_2\ \text{diff}}{HR}$$

$$O_2\ \text{Pulse} = SV \times a-\bar{v}\ O_2\ \text{diff}$$

Double Product ($M\dot{V}O_2$)

$$M\dot{V}O_2 = \frac{HR \times SBP}{100}$$

Pulse Pressure

$$\text{Pulse pressure} = SBP - DBP$$

Mean Arterial Pressure (MAP)

$$MAP = \frac{SBP - DBP}{3} + DBP$$

Pulmonary Function Calculations, Chapter 5

Air and Gas Standardization Equations

$$STPD \longleftarrow ATPS$$

$$V\ (STPD) = V\ (ATPS) \times \frac{K}{K + AT} \times \frac{P_B - P\,H_2O\ (\text{room})}{P_B}$$

$$BTPS \longleftarrow ATPS$$

$$V\ (BTPS) = V\ (ATPS) \times \frac{K + BT}{K + AT} \times \frac{P_B - P\,H_2O\ (\text{room})}{P_B - P\,H_2O\ (\text{lungs})}$$

$$BTPS \longleftarrow ATPS$$

$$V\ (STPD) = V\ (BTPS) \times \frac{K}{K + AT} \times \frac{P_B - P\,H_2O\ (\text{lung})}{P_B}$$

Minute Ventilation ($\dot{V}E$)

$$\dot{V}E = TV \times f$$

Physiological Dead Space

$$\text{Physiological DS} = \text{anatomical DS} + \text{alveolar DS}$$

Alveolar Ventilation ($\dot{V}A$)

$$\dot{V}A = \dot{V}E - (DS \times f)$$
and
$$\dot{V}A = (TV - DS) \times f$$

Oxygen Uptake ($\dot{V}O_2$)

$\dot{V}O_2 = (\dot{V}I \times FIO_2) - (\dot{V}E \times FEO_2)$ (when $\dot{V}I$ and $\dot{V}E$ are not equal)
$\dot{V}O_2 = \dot{V}E\,(FIO_2 - FEO_2)$ (when $\dot{V}I = \dot{V}E$)

Carbon Dioxide Production ($\dot{V}CO_2$)

$\dot{V}CO_2 = (\dot{V}E \times FECO_2) - (\dot{V}I \times FICO_2)$ (when $\dot{V}E$ and $\dot{V}I$ are not equal)
$\dot{V}CO_2 = \dot{V}E\,(FECO_2 - FICO_2)$ (when $\dot{V}E = \dot{V}I$)

Haldane Nitrogen Correction Equations

$$\dot{V}I = \frac{\dot{V}E \times FEN_2}{FIN_2}$$
$$\dot{V}E = \frac{\dot{V}I \times FIN_2}{VEN_2}$$
$$FIN_2 = 1.00 - FIO_2 - FICO_2$$
$$FEN_2 = 1.00 - FEO_2 - FECO_2$$

Converting Absolute $\dot{V}O_2$ to Relative $\dot{V}O_2$

$$\frac{\text{Absolute } \dot{V}O_2 \text{ in ml } O_2/\text{min}}{\text{wt of subject in kg}} = \text{Relative } \dot{V}O_2 \text{ in ml } O_2/\text{kg}/\text{min}$$

wt of subject (kg) =

Resting Energy Expenditure, Bayes Theorem, Chapter 6

REE for Males

$$\frac{\text{kcal}}{24\text{ hr}} = [66.473 + (13.752 \times \text{wt}) + (5.003 \times \text{ht})] - (6.755 \times \text{age})$$

REE for Females

$$\frac{\text{kcal}}{24\text{ hr}} = [655.096 + (9.563 \times \text{wt}) + (1.85 \times \text{ht})] - (4.676 \times \text{age})$$

Sensitivity

Used with graded exercise tests to detect heart disease among those who really have heart disease

$$\text{Sensitivity} = \frac{\text{number of positive tests}}{\text{number of positive tests} + \text{number of negative tests}} \times 100$$

Specificity

Used with graded exercise tests to detect healthy subjects among healthy subjects

$$\text{Specificity} = \frac{\text{number of negative tests}}{\text{number of negative tests} + \text{number of false positive tests}} \times 100$$

Bayes Theorem Algorithm

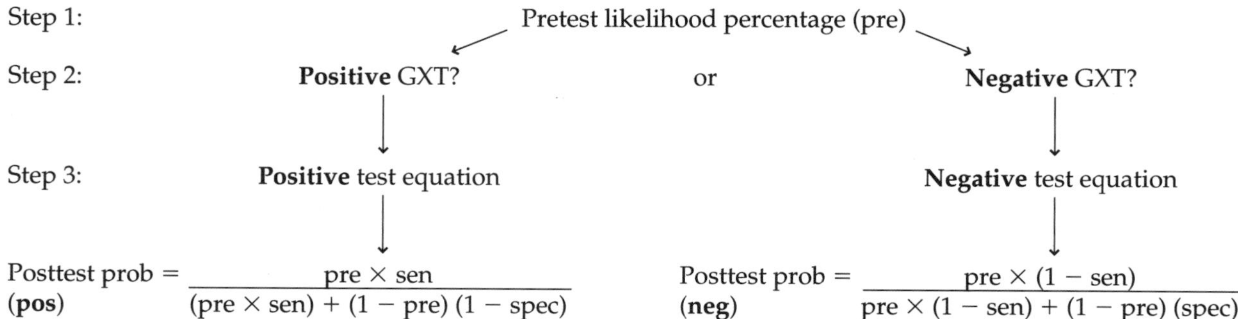

Karvonen Formula to Calculate THR

HRmax can be the highest heart rate achieved on a graded exercise test or calculated by age prediction; 220 − age = HRmax.

An example: HRmax = 195; resting HR = 55; prescribed range 70%–85%

HRmax	195
HR Rest	− 55
	140 bt/min

Lower end of training HR	Upper end of training HR
140 bt/min × .70 = 98	140 bt/min × .85 = 119
Add resting + 55	Add resting + 55
153 bt/min	174 bt/min

Training HR = 153 bt/min to 174 bt/min

Level Walking, Chapter 7

Solving for Total $\dot{V}O_2$

$$\text{Total } \dot{V}O_2 = \text{horiz } \dot{V}O_2 \text{ component} + \text{rest } \dot{V}O_2 \text{ component}$$

$$\text{Total } \dot{V}O_2 = \left(\text{speed m/min} \times \frac{0.1 \text{ ml } O_2/\text{kg/min}}{\text{m/min}}\right) + (3.5 \text{ ml } O_2/\text{kg/min})$$

Solving for Speed m/min

(First subtract 3.5 ml O_2/kg/min from the total $\dot{V}O_2$.)

$$\dot{V}O_2 \times \frac{1\ \text{m/min}}{0.1\ \text{ml}\ O_2/\text{kg/min}} = \text{speed in m/min}$$

Level and Percent Grade Walking, Chapter 8

The Complete Walking Equation

$$\text{Horiz}\ \dot{V}O_2 = \text{m/min} \times \frac{0.1\ \text{ml}\ O_2/\text{kg/min}}{\text{m/min}}$$

$$\text{Vert}\ \dot{V}O_2 = \%\ \text{grade} \times \text{m/min} \times \frac{1.8\ \text{ml}\ O_2/\text{kg/min}}{\text{m/min}}$$

$$\underline{+\ \text{Rest}\ \dot{V}O_2} = 3.5\ \text{ml}\ O_2/\text{kg/min}$$

$$\text{Total}\ \dot{V}O_2\ (\text{ml}\ O_2/\text{kg/min})$$

Level and Percent Grade Running, Chapter 9

The Complete Running Equation

$$\text{Horiz}\ \dot{V}O_2 = \text{m/min} \times \frac{0.2\ \text{ml}\ O_2/\text{kg/min}}{\text{m/min}}$$

$$\text{Vert}\ \dot{V}O_2 = \%\ \text{grade} \times \text{m/min} \times \frac{0.9\ \text{ml}\ O_2/\text{kg/min}}{\text{m/min}}$$

$$\underline{+\ \text{Rest}\ \dot{V}O_2} = 3.5\ \text{ml}\ O_2/\text{kg/min}$$

$$\text{Total}\ \dot{V}O_2\ (\text{ml}\ O_2/\text{kg/min})$$

Cycle and Arm Ergometer Equations, Chapter 10

The Complete Cycle Equation

$$\text{Vert}\ \dot{V}O_2 = \frac{\text{kgm}}{\text{min}} \times \frac{2\ \text{ml}\ O_2}{\text{kgm}}$$

$$+\ \underline{\text{Rest}\ \dot{V}O_2} = \frac{3.5\ \text{ml}\ O_2}{\text{kg/min}} \times \frac{\text{kg body wt}}{1}$$

$$\text{Total}\ \dot{V}O_2\ (\text{ml}\ O_2/\text{min})$$

Solving for kgm/min Workload for Cycle

(First subtract the rest $\dot{V}O_2$ from the total $\dot{V}O_2$.)

$$\dot{V}O_2 \times \frac{\text{kgm}}{2\ \text{ml}\ O_2} = \text{kgm/min workload}$$

Solving for Pedal Resistance in kg of Drag for Arm and Cycle Ergometer

$$\text{Kg resistance} = \frac{\text{kgm}}{\text{min}} \times \frac{\text{rev}}{\text{m}} \times \frac{\text{min}}{\text{rev}}$$

The Complete Arm Crank Ergometer Equation

$$\begin{aligned} \text{Resistive } \dot{V}O_2 &= \frac{\text{kgm}}{\text{min}} \times \frac{3 \text{ ml } O_2}{\text{kgm}} \\ \underline{+ \text{ Rest } \dot{V}O_2} &= \frac{3.5 \text{ ml } O_2}{\text{kg/min}} \times \frac{\text{kg body wt}}{1} \\ \text{Total } \dot{V}O_2 \text{ (ml } O_2\text{/min)} & \end{aligned}$$

Solving for kgm/min Workload for Arm Ergometer

(First subtract the rest $\dot{V}O_2$ from the total $\dot{V}O_2$.)

$$\dot{V}O_2 \times \frac{\text{kgm}}{3 \text{ ml } O_2} = \text{kgm/min workload}$$

Calculations for Bench Stepping, Chapter 11

The Complete Bench Stepping Equation

$$\begin{aligned} \text{Horiz } \dot{V}O_2 &= \frac{\text{step}}{\text{min}} \times \frac{0.35 \text{ ml } O_2\text{/kg/min}}{\text{step/min}} \\ \underline{+ \text{ Vert } \dot{V}O_2} &= \frac{\text{m}}{\text{step}} \times \frac{\text{step}}{\text{min}} \times \frac{2.4 \text{ ml } O_2\text{/kg/min}}{\text{m/min}} \\ \text{Total } \dot{V}O_2 \text{ (ml } O_2\text{/kg/min)} & \end{aligned}$$

Submaximal Exercise Testing and Related Math, Chapter 12

McArdle's Three-Minute Step Test

$\dot{V}O_2\text{max (males)} = 111.33 - (0.42 \times HR)$ — A 3-min test at 24 step cycles/min

$\dot{V}O_2\text{max (females)} = 65.81 - (0.1847 \times HR)$ — A 3-min test at 22 step cycles/min

Mahar's Single HR-$\dot{V}O_2$ Equation to Estimate $\dot{V}O_2max$

$$\text{Men: Est } \dot{V}O_2\text{max} = \text{final } \dot{V}O_2 \times \left(\frac{\text{HRmax} - 61}{\text{Final HR} - 61}\right)$$

$$\text{Women: Est } \dot{V}O_2\text{max} = \text{final } \dot{V}O_2 \times \left(\frac{\text{HRmax} - 72}{\text{Final HR} - 72}\right)$$

Shepherd's Double HR-$\dot{V}O_2$ Equation to Estimate $\dot{V}O_2max$

$$\dot{V}O_2max = 2nd\ \dot{V}O_2 + \left[\left(\frac{2nd\ \dot{V}O_2 - 1st\ \dot{V}O_2}{2nd\ HR - 1st\ HR}\right) \times (HRmax - 2nd\ HR)\right]$$

Pollock's THR-$\dot{V}O_2$ Equation to Estimate $\dot{V}O_2max$

$$Est\ \dot{V}O_2max = final\ \dot{V}O_2 \times 1.174$$

Nutrition Math, Chapter 13

See Appendix B for conversion factors for protein, carb, and fat to kcal.

Calculating Protein Requirements

$$kg\ ideal\ body\ wt \times \frac{.8\ g\ protein}{1\ kg\ body\ wt} = g\ protein\ required\ per\ day$$

Protein requirements can also be determined using a subject's total body weight.

Respiratory Quotient (RQ) and Respiratory Gas Exchange Rate (R)

$$RQ = R = \frac{VCO_2}{VO_2}$$

Glossary

absolute $\dot{V}O_2$—The amount of oxygen consumption in 1 min, expressed in the units ml O_2/min.

alveolar ventilation ($\dot{V}A$)—The volume of air that reaches the alveoli of the lungs during each minute at rest or during exercise.

anaerobic threshold—A demarcation point between moderate and intense exercise. At this point CO_2 production, minute ventilation, and blood levels of lactic acid begin to increase sharply.

arteriovenous O_2 difference (a-$\bar{v}$ O_2 diff)—The difference in oxygen content between arterial and mixed venous blood.

ATPS—A gas volume that is at ambient temperature and pressure and is saturated with water.

basal metabolic rate (BMR)—Energy metabolism that is sufficient only to support the resting state.

Bayesian analysis—A method of determining the likelihood of coronary heart disease based upon symptoms before a graded exercise test and ECG ischemic response during a graded exercise test.

BTPS—A gas volume that is at body temperature and ambient pressure and is saturated with water.

Calorie (kcal)—The amount of energy that can raise 1 kg of water 1 °Celsius. Calorie is the term used to measure the energy contained in foods.

carbohydrate—One of the three energy nutrients; contains 4 kcal/g.

cardiac output ($\dot{Q}$)—The volume of blood pumped by the left ventricle per heartbeat per minute (ml blood/bt).

cardiac reserve—A measure of the heart's ability to increase its cardiac output ($\dot{Q}$) from rest up to maximal exercise, which is the difference between $\dot{Q}$ at rest and $\dot{Q}$ at maximal exercise.

cholesterol—A type of lipid (fat) that is manufactured within the body as well as derived from foods that come from animal products. This type of lipid is part of every body cell structure and most hormones. Only when in excess does cholesterol contribute to plaque formation within arteries.

conversion factor—A mathematical tool written in the form of a fraction that facilitates changing one unit to another unit without changing the value of the number.

dead space—The volume of air within the respiratory system that is not involved in gas exchange.

diastole—The resting or filling period of the heart's cardiac cycle.

diastolic blood pressure—Arterial pressure (mmHg) during the resting or filling period of the heart's cardiac cycle.

double product—Also known as the rate-pressure product; the product of heart rate × systolic blood pressure, indicating the heart's oxygen requirement at the time of ECG ischemic ST wave depression or angina symptoms occur.

ejection fraction (EF)—The percentage of blood that is pumped out of the left ventricle compared to the volume of blood that remains after the systolic beat. EF = stroke volume/end diastolic volume.

electrocardiogram (ECG or EKG)—A recording of the electrical activity of the heart.

end diastolic volume (EDV)—The volume of blood that remains in the left ventricle at the end of cardiac diastole.

end systolic volume (ESV)—The volume of blood that remains in the left ventricle after the systolic beat.

ergometer—Any piece of exercise equipment that has an accurate indicator of workloads.

exercise—A single session of energy expenditure above rest.

fat—An energy nutrient that contains 9 kcal/g.

Fick equation—Cardiac output × arteriovenous oxygen difference = $\dot{V}O_2$.

fitness—Positive physiological adaptations as a result of a series of exercise sessions.

Frank-Starling law—A principle stating that stroke volume (SV) increases in response to heart muscle stretch during diastolic filling.

graded exercise test (GXT)—An evaluation of fitness, using a system of progressive workloads, that can be performed using any ergometer.

heart rate (HR)—The number of heartbeats in 1 min (bt/min).

heart rate reserve—A measure of the heart's ability to increase its rate from rest up to maximal exercise.

high density lipoprotein (HDL)—A fraction of total cholesterol that is a protective component for heart disease.

ideal body weight (IBW)—Total body weight for adults; allows a subject to be within a healthy range for percentage of body fat.

intensity—The level of effort put forth during exercise; measured in METs (metabolic equivalents).

kilocalorie (kcal)—A measure of energy stored in foods. One kcal can raise 1 kg of water from 0 °C up to 1 °C.

kilogram-meter/min—A unit of work in which a gram of weight is moved straight up to a distance of 1 m within 1 min, abbreviated kgm/min. The cycle and arm ergometer use the kgm/min as a unit of work.

lean body weight—The portion of total body weight that is non-fat, composed of muscle, bones, fluids, tendons, ligaments, and other protein and connective tissues.

lipids—A general term referring to the fatty substances that are carried through the blood stream.

lipoprotein—A molecule made up of protein and a fat.

low density lipoprotein (LDL)—A molecule responsible for transport of cholesterol through the blood stream. LDL deposits excess cholesterol onto the walls of the arterial system. High plasma levels of LDL are a major risk factor for heart disease.

maximal heart rate (HRmax)—The highest heart rate that a subject can achieve during a graded exercise test. The HRmax can also be estimated by subtracting age from an HR of 220 bt/min.

maximal oxygen uptake ($\dot{V}O_2$max)—The greatest amount of oxygen that can be consumed on a given ergometer despite increasing workloads and continued effort by the subject. At this point, although workloads increase, oxygen uptake levels off or plateaus.

MET—Metabolic equivalent. One MET equals 3.5 ml O_2/kg/min. When you are sitting at rest you are expending the energy equivalent to one MET.

metabolism—The sum total of energy expended and created.

minute ventilation ($\dot{V}E$)—The volume of air expired in 1 min.

myocardiac infarction (MI)—Also known as heart attack; an area of heart muscle tissue dies because of lack of oxygenated blood supply.

oxygen consumption—Volume and rate at which the body consumes oxygen.

peak heart rate—The highest heart rate achieved during a graded exercise test.

peak $\dot{V}O_2$—The highest volume of oxygen consumption achieved during a graded exercise test.

predicted maximal heart rate—An estimation of HRmax; calculated by subtracting age from a heart rate of 220 bt/min.

protein—An energy nutrient that contains 4 kcal/g.

rate-pressure product—Also known as double product; the product of systolic blood pressure and heart rate. See double product.

rating of perceived exertion scale (RPE)—A scale used to help identify a subject's intensity of effort during exercise or during a graded exercise test. There are two of these scales. The scale of 1-20, with 20 representing total exhaustion, is the original scale. The second scale, 1-10, is most often used during graded exercise tests when a subject is wearing a mouthpiece. The 10 in this scale represents total exhaustion.

recommended dietary allowance (RDA)—The advised level of intake, on a daily average over several days, of specified nutrients.

relative $\dot{V}O_2$—The volume of oxygen consumed per minute in relationship to a subject's body weight in kilograms, expressed as ml O_2/kg/min.

respiratory gas exchange ratio (R)—A reflection of the ratio of CO_2 production and O_2 consumption at the lung level. An R of greater than 1.00 is one of the indicators of $\dot{V}O_2$max.

respiratory quotient (RQ)—The ratio of CO_2 production to O_2 consumption at the cellular level at rest or during steady-state submaximal exercise; an indicator of food source metabolism.

rest—One MET, which is a state of resting metabolism characterized by the relative oxygen consumption of 3.5 ml O_2/kg/min.

sensitivity—An indicator of the ability of a graded exercise test to detect heart disease in a group of subjects who all really do have heart disease.

specificity—An indicator of the ability of a graded exercise test to detect healthy subjects when all subjects are truly healthy.

STPD—A gas volume that is at standard temperature and pressure and is dry of water vapor. Standard conditions are 0 °C, a pressure of 760 mmHg (standard atmosphere), and no water vapor in the gas volume.

stroke volume (SV)—The volume of blood pumped (ejected) by either ventricle during one heartbeat.

ST segment depression—An ECG change that reflects myocardiac ischemia, characterized by the ST segment dropping 1 to 2 mm below (or sometime rising above) the ECG isoelectric baseline.

submaximal—Related to exercise intensity whereby the heart rate is below 85% of HRmax.

systole—The contraction phase of the cardiac cycle.

systolic blood pressure—Arterial pressure during the contraction phase of the cardiac cycle, measured in mmHg (millimeters of mercury).

target heart rate (THR)—The stopping heart rate used during a submaximal exercise test. The target heart rate is usually 85% of 220 − age.

tidal volume (TV)—Volume of air that is inhaled or exhaled with each breath.

training heart rate (THR)—A heart rate range that is about 60% to 85% of HRmax; a range that is most efficient for improving aerobic power.

triglycerides—Stored free fatty acids within adipose tissue; also used as a source of energy. Elevated triglycerides are a contributing factor for heart disease.

unit of measure (unit)—A term used to label a number. As an example, in the value of 68 kg, the 68 is the number and the kg is the unit. The unit gives meaning to the number.

$\dot{V}O_2$max—See maximal oxygen consumption.

volume—The measure of the quantity of a substance. In this book we are concerned with the volume of oxygen, volume of air, and volume of blood. Liters (L) or milliliters (ml) are units of measure used to label a volume.

Bibliography

Adamovich, D. R. (1984). *The heart.* Newell, Iowa: Bireline.

Adams, W. C. (1967). Influence of age, sex and body weight on the energy expenditure of cycle riding. *Journal of Applied Physiology,* **22,** 539–545.

American College of Sports Medicine. (1988). *Resource Manual For Guidelines For Exercise Testing and Prescription.* Philadelphia: Lea & Febiger.

American College of Sports Medicine. (1995). *Guidelines for Exercise Testing and Prescription* (5th ed.). Philadelphia: Lea & Febiger.

American Heart Association. (1974). *Exercise testing and training of apparently healthy individuals: A handbook for physicians.* New York, NY: Author. (Committee on Exercise)

American Heart Association. (1982, September-October; November-December). Rationale of the diet-heart statement of the American Heart Association. *Nutrition Today,* pp. 16–20; 15–19. (Committee report)

American Heart Association. (1988). Dietary guidelines for healthy American adults: A statement for physicians and health professionals by the Nutrition Committee, American Heart Association. *Circulation,* **77,** 721A–724A.

Astrand, P.-O., & Rodahl, K. (1986). *Textbook of Work Physiology* (3rd ed.). New York: McGraw-Hill.

Balke, B. (1959). An experimental study of physical fitness of Air Force personnel. *US Armed Forces Medical Journal,* **10,** 675–688.

Berry, M. J., Storsteen, J. A., & Woodard, C. M. (1993). Effects of body mass on exercise efficiency and $\dot{V}O_2$ during steady-state cycling. *Medicine and Science in Sports and Exercise,* **25,** 1031–1037.

Bevegard, B. S. (1966). Circulatory adaptation to arm and leg exercise in supine and sitting position. *Journal of Applied Physiology,* **21,** 37–46.

Bevegard, B. S., & Shepard, J. (1967). Regulation of circulation during exercise in man. *Physiological Reviews,* **47,** 178–213.

Borg, G. A. V. (1982). Psychological bases of physical exertion. *Medicine and Science in Sports and Exercise,* **14,** 377–381.

Bouchard, C., Shephard, R. J., Stephens, T., Sutton, J. R., & McPherson, B. D. (Eds.) (1990). *Exercise, fitness, and health: A consensus of current knowledge.* Champaign, IL: Human Kinetics.

Brooks, G. A. (1985). Anerobic threshold: Review of the concept and directions for future research. *Medicine and Science in Sports and Exercise,* **17,** 22–31.

Brooks, G. A., & Fahey, T. D. (1984). *Exercise physiology, human bioenergetics and its applications.* New York: Wiley.

Brown, M. S., & Goldstein, J. L. (1986). A receptor-mediated pathway for cholesterol homeostasis. *Science,* **232,** 34–47.

Bruce, R. A. (1973). Maximal oxygen intake and nomographic assessment of functional aerobic impairment in cardiovascular disease. *American Heart Journal,* **85,** 546–562.

Bruce, R. A. (1974). Separation of effects of CVD and age on ventricular function with maximal exercise. *American Journal of Cardiology,* **34,** 757–769.

Bruce, R. A. (1977). Exercise testing for evaluation of ventricular function. *New England Journal of Medicine,* **296,** 671–675.

Coleman, A. E. (1976). Validation of a submaximal test of maximal oxygen intake. *Journal of Sports Medicine and Physical Fitness,* **16,** 106–111.

Cooper, K. H. (1968). A means of assessing maximal oxygen intake. Correlation between field and treadmill testing. *Journal of the American Medical Association,* **203,** 201–204.

Davies, K., Packer, L., & Brooks, G. A. (1981). Biochemical adaptation of mitochondria, muscle and whole animal respiration to endurance training. *Archives of Biochemistry and Biophysics,* **209,** 539–554.

Davis, J. A. (1985). Anaerobic threshold: Review of the concept and directions for future research. *Medicine and Science in Sports and Exercise,* **17,** 6–18.

deVries, H. A. (1986). *Physiology of Exercise.* Dubuque, IA: Brown.

Diamond, G. A., & Forrester, J. S. (1979). Analysis of probability as an aid in the clinical diagnosis of coronary-artery disease. *New England Journal of Medicine,* **300,** 1350–1358.

Dill, D. B. (1965). Oxygen used in horizontal and grade walking and running on the treadmill. *Journal of Applied Physiology,* **20,** 19–22.

Dissik, J. (1972). Production of gaseous nitrogen in human steady state conditions. *Journal of Applied Physiology,* **32,** 155–159.

Donovan, C. M., & Brooks, G. A. (1977). Muscular efficiency during steady-state exercise. Effects of walking speed and work rate. *Journal of Applied Physiology,* **43,** 431–439.

Ellestad, M. H. (1986). *Stress testing.* Philadelphia: Davis.

Epstein, S. E. (1979). Limitations of electrocardiographic exercise testing. *New England Journal of Medicine,* **301,** 264–265.

Epstein, S. E. (1980). Implications of probability analysis on the strategy used for noninvasive detection of coronary artery disease. *American Journal of Cardiology,* **46,** 491–499.

Fardy, P. (1977). Benefits of arm exercise in cardiac rehabilitation. *Physiology of Sports Medicine,* **5,** 31–41.

Farrell, S. W., Ivy, J. L. (1987). Lactate acidosis and the increase in $\dot{V}E/\dot{V}O_2$ during incremental exercise. *Journal of Applied Physiology,* **62,** 1551–1555.

Fleming, J. K. (1990). Cholesterol: The good, the bad and the confusing. *Roche Testrends,* **4**(3), 2–4.

Fletcher, G. (1988). *Exercise in the practice of medicine.* Mount Kisco, NY: Futura.

Foster, C. (1984). Generalized equations for predicting functional capacity from treadmill performance. *American Heart Journal,* **107,** 1229–1235.

Fox, E. L. (1973). A simple accurate technique for predicting maximal aerobic power. *Journal of Applied Physiology,* **35,** 914.

Fox, E. L., Bowers, R. W., & Foss, M. L. (1988). *The physiological basis of physical education and athletics.* New York: Saunders.

Franklin, B. A. (1982a). Arm exercise testing and training. *Practical Cardiology,* **8,** 43–70.

Franklin, B. A. (1982b). The "MET" concept in exercise testing and prescription. *Health Care Quarterly Review,* **1,** 14–16.

Franklin, B. A. (1983). Aerobic requirements of arm ergometry: Implications for exercise testing and training. *Physiology of Sports Medicine,* **11,** 81–90.

Franklin, B. A., Gordon, S., & Timmis, G. C. (Eds.) (1989). *Exercise in modern medicine.* Baltimore: Williams & Wilkins.

Franklin, B. A., Vander, L., Wrisley, D., & Rubenfire, M. (1983). Aerobic requirements of arm ergometry: Implications of exercise testing and training. *Physiology of Sports Medicine,* **11,** 81–90.

Froelicher, V. F. (1973). The correlation of coronary angiography and the electrocardiographic response to maximal treadmill testing in 76 asymptomatic men. *Circulation,* **48,** 597–604.

Froelicher, V. F. (1975). Prediction of maximal oxygen consumption: Comparison of the Bruce and Balke treadmill protocols. *Chest,* **68,** 331–336.

Froelicher, V. F. (1987). *Exercise and the heart.* Chicago: Year Book Medical.

Froelicher, V. F. (1989). *Manual of exercise testing.* Chicago: Year Book Medical.

Glass, G. (1984). *Statistical methods in education and psychology.* Englewood Cliffs, NJ: Prentice Hall.

Goldberg, L., & Elliot, D. L. (1985). The effects of physical activity on lipids and lipoprotein levels. *Medical Clinics of North America,* **69,** 41–55.

Goldberger, A. L. (1991). *Myocardial infarction.* St. Louis: Mosby.

Golding, L. A., Myers, C. R., & Sinning, W. E. (1982). *The Y's way to physical fitness: A guidebook for instructors.* Champaign, IL: Human Kinetics.

Golding, L. A., Myers, C. R., & Sinning, W. E. (1989). *The Y's way to physical fitness: A complete guide to fitness testing and instruction* (3rd ed.). Champaign, IL: Human Kinetics.

Griner, P. (1980). Selection and interpretation of diagnostic tests and procedures: Principles and application. *Annals of Internal Medicine,* **94,** 553–600.

Guyton, A. C. (1991). *Textbook of medical physiology* (8th ed.). Philadelphia: Saunders.

Hellerstein, H. K. (1984). *Rehabilitation of the coronary patient.* New York: Wiley.

Heyward, V. H. (1991). *Advanced fitness assessment and exercise prescription.* Champaign, IL: Human Kinetics.

Howley, E. T., & Franks, B. D. (1992). *Health fitness instructor's handbook.* Champaign, IL: Human Kinetics.

Johnson, R., Brouha, L., & Darling, C. (1942). A test of physical fitness for strenuous exertion. *Review of Canadian Biology,* **1,** 491.

Jones, N. L. (1988). *Clinical exercise testing.* Philadelphia: Saunders.

Jones, R. H. (1981). Accuracy of diagnosis of coronary artery disease by radionuclide measurement of left ventricular function during rest and exercise. *Circulation,* **64,** 585–601.

Kasch, F. W., Phillips, W., Ross, D., Carter, L., & Boyer, J. L. (1966). A comparison of maximal oxygen uptake by treadmill and step-test procedures. *Journal of Applied Physiology,* **21,** 1387.

Katch, F. I. (1973). Relationship between individual differences in steady-pace endurance running performance and maximal oxygen uptake. *Research Quarterly for Exercise and Sport,* **44,** 206.

Langler, L. L. (1971). *Review of physiology.* New York: McGraw-Hill.

Latin, R. W., Berg, K. E., Smith, P., Tolle, R., & Woodby-Brown, S. (1993). Validation of a cycle ergometer equation for predicting steady-rate $\dot{V}O_2$. *Medicine and Science in Sports and Exercise,* **25,** 970–974.

Leverton, R. M. (1975). The RDAs are not for amateurs. *Journal of the American Dietetic Association,* **66,** 9–11.

Lohman, T. G. (1981). Skinfolds and body density and their relation to body fatness, a review. *Human Biology,* **53,** 181–225.

Lohman, T. G. (1984a). Preface to body composition assessment: A re-evaluation of our past and a look toward the future. *Medicine and Science in Sports and Exercise,* **16,** 578.

Lohman, T. G. (1984b). Research progress in validation of laboratory methods of assessing body composition. *Medicine and Science in Sports and Exercise,* **16,** 596–603.

Mahar, M. (1985). Predictive accuracy of single and double stage submax treadmill work for estimating aerobic capacity. *Medicine and Science in Sports and Exercise,* **17,** 206–207.

Marable, N. L. (1979). Urinary nitrogen excretion as influenced by a muscle-building exercise program and protein intake variation. *Nutrition Reports International,* **19,** 795–805.

Margaria, R., Cerretelli, P., & Aghemo, P. (1963). Energy cost of running. *Journal of Applied Physiology,* **18,** 367–379.

Master, A., Prody, L., & Chesky, K. (1953). Two-step exercise electrocardiogram. *Journal of the American Medical Association,* **151,** 458.

McArdle, W. D., Katch, F. I., & Katch, V. L. (1994). *Exercise physiology: Energy, nutrition and human Performance* (4th ed.). Philadelphia: Lea & Febiger.

McArdle, W. D., Katch, F. I., Pechar, G. S., Jacobson, L., & Ruck, S. (1972). Reliability and interrelationships between maximal oxygen intake, physical working capacity and step-test scores in college women. *Medicine and Science in Sport and Exercise,* **4,** 182–186.

McLellan, T. (1992). A comparative evaluation of the individual anaerobic threshold and critical power. *Medicine and Science in Sports and Exercise,* **24,** 543–550.

Mitchell, J. H. (1992). How to recognize "athlete's heart." *Physiology of Sports Medicine,* **20,** 87–96.

Motil, K. (1990). Dietary protein and nitrogen balance in lactating and non-lactating women. *American Journal of Clinical Nutrition,* **51,** 378–384.

Nagle, F. J., Balke, B., & Naughton, F. P. (1965). Gradational step test for assessing work capacity. *Journal of Applied Physiology,* **20,** 745–748.

National Institutes of Health. (1984). Treatment of hypertriglyceremia: Consensus conference. *Journal of the American Medical Association,* **251,** 1196–1200.

National Research Council. (1989). *Diet and health: Implications for reducing chronic disease risk.* Washington, DC: National Academy Press.

Nunn, J. (1987). *Applied respiratory physiology.* London: Butterworth.

Passmore, R., & Durnin, J. V. G. A. (1955). Human energy expenditure. *Physiological Review,* **35,** 801–840.

Poliner, L. R. (1980). Left ventricle performance in normal subjects. *Circulation,* **62,** 528–534.

Pollock, M. L. (1976). A comparative analysis of four protocols for maximal treadmill stress testing. *American Heart Journal,* **92,** 39–46.

Pollock, M. L., Wilmore, J. H., & Fox, S. M. (1978). *Health and fitness through physical activity.* New York: Wiley.

Pollock, M. L., Wilmore, J. H., & Fox, S. M. (1984). *Exercise in health and disease.* Philadelphia: Saunders.

Powers, S. K., & Howley, E. T. (1990). *Exercise physiology: Theory and application to fitness and performance.* Dubuque, IA: Brown.

Pulsinelli, L. R., & Hooper, P. I. (1987). *Introductory algebra: An interactive approach.* New York: Macmillan.

Rifkin, R. D., & Hood, W. B. (1977). Bayesian analysis of electrocardiographic exercise stress testing. *New England Journal of Medicine,* **297,** 681–86.

Runyon, R. (1976). *Fundamentals of behavioral statistics.* Menlo Park, CA: Addison-Wesley.

Ruppel, G. (1991). *Manual of pulmonary function testing.* St. Louis: Mosby.

Rusko, H., Havu, M., & Karvinen, E. (1978). Aerobic performance capacity in athletes. *European Journal of Applied Physiology,* **38,** 151–159.

Saltin, B., Astrand, P.-O. (1967). Maximal oxygen uptake in athletes. *Journal of Applied Physiology,* **23,** 353.

Sharkey, B. J. (1991). *New dimensions in aerobic fitness* (Monograph no. 1). Champaign, IL: Human Kinetics.

Shephard, R. S. (1970). Computer programs for solution of Astrand nomogram and the calculation of body surface area. *Journal of Sports Medicine and Physical Fitness,* **10,** 206–210.

Shephard, R. S. (1972). *Alive man: The physiology of physical activity.* Springfield, IL: Charles C Thomas.

Shephard, R. S. (1984). Tests of maximum oxygen intake: A critical review. *Sports Medicine,* **1,** 99–124.

Skidmore-Roth, L. (1992). *Mosby's nursing drug reference.* St. Louis: Mosby.

Skinner, J. (1985). Submaximal endurance performance elated to ventilation thresholds. *Canadian Journal of Applied Sport Science,* **10,** 81–87.

Sox, H. (1988). *Medical decision making.* Boston: Butterworth.

Sox, H. (1990). *Common Diagnostic Tests.* Philadelphia: American College of Physicians.

Strauss, R. H. (1979). *Sports Medicine and Physiology.* Philadelphia: Saunders.

Toner, M. M., Glickman, E. L., & McArdle, W. D. (1990). Cardiovascular adjustments to exercise distributed between the upper and lower body. *Medicine and Science in Sports and Exercise,* **22,** 773–778.

Torg, J. S., Welsh, R, P., & Shephard, R. J. (1990). *Current therapy in sports medicine - 2.* Philadelphia: Decker.

Vander, A. J., Sherman, J. H., & Luciano, D. S. (1975). *Human physiology.* New York: McGraw-Hill.

Van-der Walt, W. H., & Wyndham, C. H. (1973). An equation for prediction of energy expenditure of walking and running. *Journal of Applied Physiology,* **34,** 559.

Wasserman, K., Hansen, J. E., Sue, D. Y., & Whipp, B. J. (1987). *Principles of exercise testing and interpretation.* Philadelphia: Lea & Febiger.

Weiner, D. A., Thomas, J. R., McCabe, C. H., Kennedy, J. W., Schloss, M., Tristani, F., Chaitman, B. R., & Fisher, L D. (1979). Exercise stress testing. Correlations among history of angina, ST-segment response and prevalence of coronary-artery disease in the coronary artery surgery study. *New England Journal of Medicine,* **301,** 230–235.

Weinstein, M. (1980). *Clinical decision analysis.* Philadelphia: Saunders.

Whitney, E. N., & Hamilton, E. M. N. (1977). *Understanding nutrition.* New York: West.

Wilmore, J. H. (1982). *Training for sport and activity.* Boston: Allyn & Bacon.

Worthington-Roberts, B. S. (1981). *Contemporary developments in Nutrition.* St. Louis: Mosby.

Zavala, D. (1987). *Manual on exercise testing, a training handbook.* Iowa City, IA: University of Iowa.

Zavala, D. C. (1989). *Nutritional assessment in critical care.* Iowa City, IA: University of Iowa.

Index

R

S

T

About the Author

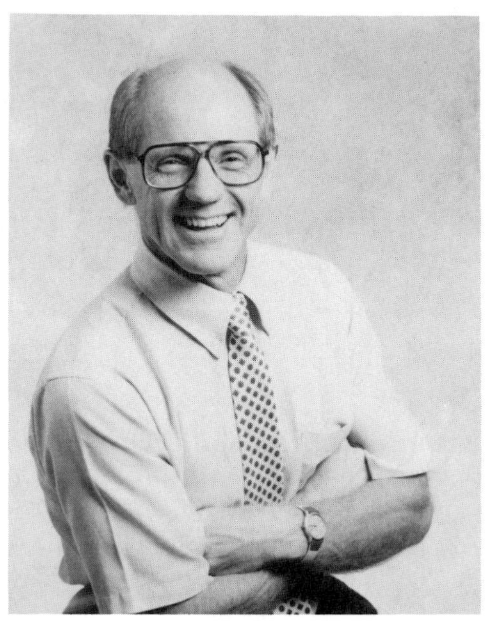

Dennis K. Flood began his career in exercise physiology at The Cooper Institute for Aerobics Research in Dallas, Texas, conducting stress testing in the Strength Lab. After working in cardiac rehabilitation at Presbyterian Hospital in Dallas and All-Saints Hospital in Fort Worth, Dennis became manager of cardiac rehabilitation at Campbell Hospital in Weatherford, Texas, where he helped develop a highly successful program for adult fitness, employee fitness, and Phase I, II, and III cardiac rehabilitation. Later, Flood was manager of the cardiac rehabilitation program at HCA Lewisville Hospital in Lewisville, Texas. Today he is the director of Sports Medicine, Cardiac Rehab, and Employee Fitness/Wellness at Sarasota Memorial Hospital in Sarasota, Florida.

Flood received an MS in exercise physiology from North Texas State University in 1988. He is certified by the American College of Sports Medicine (ACSM) as an exercise test technologist, the American Council on Exercise as a personal trainer, and the American Heart Association in advanced cardiac life support. He is a member of ACSM and the American Association of Cardiovascular and Pulmonary Rehabilitation. In his free time, Flood enjoys sailing, running, cycling, swimming in the ocean, competing in triathlons, and surfing.